How to Get Pregnant

HARRIET GRIFFEY is a freelance print and broadcast journalist who writes regularly for UK national newspapers and magazines. She originally trained as a nurse at the Middlesex Hospital, London but subsequently worked in book publishing, television, radio and journalism. She is the author of numerous books including *The Really Useful A–Z of Pregnancy & Birth*, *The Art of the Nap*, *Boost Your Child's Immune System* and *The Art of Concentration*. She has two sons and lives in London. www.harrietgriffey.com

How to Get Pregnant

New Edition – Revised and Updated

HARRIET GRIFFEY

BLOOMSBURY
LONDON · BERLIN · NEW YORK · SYDNEY

First published in 1997
This revised edition published 2010

Bloomsbury Publishing Plc, 36 Soho Square, London, W1D 3QY

A CIP catalogue record for this book
is available from the British Library

ISBN 9781408808955

10 9 8 7 6 5 4 3 2 1

Designed by Neysa Moss
Typeset by Hewer Text Ltd, Edinburgh
Printed in Great Britain by Clays Ltd, St Ives plc

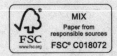

www.bloomsbury.com

Author's acknowledgements

Many people have been helpful in the writing of this book and particular thanks are due to Susan Rice at ISSUE, the National Fertility Association; Clare Lewis Jones at the Infertility Network UK; Sandra Dill of ACCESS; Tamsin May at NIAC; the late Dr Anna Flynn; Dr Rachel Pettigrew at the Assisted Conception Unit, St Thomas' Hospital, London; Belinda Barnes at Foresight; and to Emma Dally at the National Magazine Company. While their support and comments have been invaluable, the final responsibility for the book's content must rest with me.

I would also like to thank all those women and men – friends, and friends of friends – who were kind enough to share their experiences of getting pregnant, in one way or another, with me. This book is dedicated to them and to my own two children, Josh and Robbie.

Contents

1 Introduction

In the thirteen years since this book was originally published, some things have changed but one thing remains resolutely the same: there will always be some couples for whom getting pregnant is a challenge. Figures quoted by the Infertility Network UK currently put this at one in six couples. The other big change in this time is the rise in online connectivity. Never before has it been so easy to resource information and ideas, and to connect to others with similar experiences, whatever it is that links them, than now. The average age at which a woman has her first baby has also changed: many are now in their late twenties, and a much bigger proportion of women than before are delaying starting their families until their thirties and early forties. Other lifestyle factors – the long work-hours culture, fast foods, environmental pollutants – may also have contributed to the changing face of fertility in the twenty-first century.

However, it still remains that the majority of women grow up expecting to be able to have children, should they wish to. From the age at which periods begin, there is an assumption that getting pregnant can happen. In fact, once a woman begins her sexual life her main preoccupation probably will be with not getting pregnant. Over the last fifty years, as contraception became more efficient and more easily available, not only did women feel better able to avoid unwanted pregnancy, they were equally sure that getting pregnant would be possible when they wanted to. Contraception equalled choice and, it was implied, choosing to have a baby would merely be a matter of when, not if.

Equally, with more recent media coverage of the problems of infertility, a growing awareness is emerging that in spite of all the information to the contrary, such choice may not be so readily available. It may be that, having struggled to keep pregnancy at bay for so long, when choosing to try and conceive, pregnancy may not happen so easily. At this point, the promise of choice seems an empty one.

This particular dilemma is also complicated by the finite period of a woman's reproductive years – those years in which conceiving a baby is actually possible. From menarche, when periods first indicate a woman's functioning fertility cycle, to menopause, when ovulation and its attendant hormonal activity ceases. This can be between thirty to forty years, from between age ten to fifteen years old until around forty-five to fifty-five years old, depending on the individual woman. Although it seems like a long time it can pass very quickly when trying to establish a career or a relationship or both.

While age is a relevant factor, it is not the only issue when it comes to problems with conceiving. Many women encounter problems with infertility, or subfertility, and for a variety of reasons, long before age is an issue. But for those women who have delayed trying to conceive for one reason or another, their age can weigh heavy and be misconstrued as the sole reason for a problem in conceiving. What age can mean is that any contributory and even minor factor that creates a problem in conceiving can be exacerbated by being older, just because our general health and fitness tends to be less good.

An apparent inability to conceive a child when she wants can have a profound effect on a woman's view of her own femininity. It raises all sorts of questions about how a woman might view herself, her relationship and ultimately her role in life. A particular career may have been chosen because, at some later stage, it will 'fit in' with having children. Equally, to a woman in a high-powered career, having a child may be seen as an opportunity to enjoy a different pace of life. An inability to conceive may also challenge assumptions about what it means, in the society in which we live, to be a woman. For many women, having a career in some way challenges their femininity while having a baby endorses it: so in order to justify one with the other, it becomes more important to have both. Westernised society is still not really reconciled with the idea of working mothers, and still seems to apply these double standards.

All sorts of issues that may never be relevant to the woman who slips easily into pregnancy without a second thought can be difficult to accept if you are experiencing problems, even if these are only short-lived. We may never have to weigh up the pros and cons of having a baby if it just 'happens'. Then it is a question of just getting on with it. But when you feel pressure to justify your desire for a baby, because getting pregnant is not happening, then trying to have a baby can become an emotionally isolating experience.

One of the first things to stress is that very few people are actually totally infertile. Very often it can be a combination of a couple of minor factors that make conception difficult but theoretically possible. While statistics tell us that one in six couples have some problem conceiving at some time, that also means that five out of six couples do not have a problem. And if the figure of around 600,000 people currently having some form of infertility treatment sounds a lot, remember that the range of different treatments varies enormously and this does not mean that the majority will not, eventually, be successful in having a baby.

More importantly perhaps, keep the following in mind: a couple with no fertility problems still have only a one in four chance of conceiving in any one month. This is normal. And about 85–90% of couples conceive within the first year of trying, while 95% of all couples will have conceived by the end of two years. Getting pregnant just can take more time for some couples than others.

Male infertility raises slightly different issues to female infertility, although it may have similar repercussions, largely because a woman's fertility is so much more a feature of her daily life than a man's. For women, the monthly cycle of hormonal fluctuations and menstrual bleeding are a regular testament to the possibility of pregnancy. Each period tells a woman that she is functioning and *could* get pregnant, while also telling her that she *has not* got pregnant this time. For men, their fertility is less obvious. Male ejaculation occurs with orgasm, is part of a man's self-view of his virility and is inextricably linked with the idea of fertility. Such an obvious indication of his masculine potential is evident on a much more regular basis than for his partner. Yet the real potency of a man's ability to make his partner pregnant is also hidden, and only truly apparent when pregnancy occurs. If this does not happen, and the problem appears to lie with the man, it questions his masculinity in a way that is similar to a woman's questioning of her femininity. Similar feelings of self-doubt, self-blame, grief and anxiety about the future of his relationship exist for a man in this situation.

Deciding to have a baby at all is not easy. There seldom seems to be a perfect time. Career-paths can feel threatened by 'wrong' timing, which may have an impact on a couple's financial income, or the threat of job loss can contribute to general anxieties about the possibilities of financially supporting a family. The arrival of children brings with it a natural curtailment of freedom if both partners are making an equal commitment to the future raising of a family. In some cases, while one partner may be ready for this, the other may find the whole idea terrifying.

Many couples would admit that there is seldom an *ideal* time to plan a family, but the best time must be when both partners are in agreement. This tacit agreement may always have been a part of the relationship, but agreeing on the timing is not always so easy. Having decided to go ahead, actively planning to have a baby and then to find that it does not happen within the first few months can be frustrating, especially if other life decisions are linked to having a baby. These may include moving house, or staying in a job only because it is the best option if a baby comes along. These issues can become linked and an apparent delay in progress, when it affects other plans, has its own difficulties.

For those for whom getting pregnant is straightforward, or happens without planning or forethought, these issues do not necessarily arise. But for couples for whom there is a conscious decision-making process, and *then* nothing happens, it can create stress within a relationship. If this occurs at any stage it is important to try and discuss the issues as and when they arise. This is not always easy, and requires reflection, honesty and a persistent desire to try and talk things through. It can become all too easy to focus on the mechanics of trying to get pregnant, while forgetting the emotional component of wanting to have a baby, which is often the expression of love for another person.

The mechanics of making a baby are well known to us all. It all sounds so simple, but in reality the whole process is more subtle. Ask a sample of women when they are most likely to conceive and you will get a variety of answers. For most of their reproductive lives, this is information that women do not need. The blanket use of contraception and proviso that it be used on 'every conceivable occasion' means, by implication, every time they have sexual intercourse suggesting that they are fertile all the time, which is completely untrue. The first step for women who are having some trouble conceiving is to gain insight into their own fertility cycle, so that they can work out more accurately when ovulation occurs, and when conception might be possible. This book includes a whole chapter on the female fertility cycle because of the importance of understanding individual fertility cycles when trying to get pregnant.

Learning about your individual fertility cycle is a valuable exercise for a number of reasons. First, better timing of intercourse dramatically improves the chances of conception. Second, it allows a woman some feeling of continuing control over events: it is all too easy to get swept away by the apparent success of medical intervention when handing over this responsibility may not, in the long term, be the most beneficial option. Infertility investigations are extremely demanding, as is assisted conception. Third, it provides essential information about an individual woman's fertility cycle which is an extremely useful resource to have when considering any further tests and treatments a doctor may suggest. Fourth, if the quality and quantity of the man's sperm is borderline, it also improves the chances for effective fertilisation of an egg.

One couple consulted a natural family planning teacher following problems in conceiving. While the man had a known borderline sperm count, it was his wife who had been on a course of the fertility drug Clomid to boost ovulation, even though there was no apparent problem! Subsequently, the charts recording her temperature and other signs of fertility showed, as she thought, that she was ovulating regularly and normally. Within a couple of months following consultation, the couple had conceived normally in spite of the man's borderline sperm count and without medical intervention.

Feeling confident about the ability to conceive is easily knocked as time passes or reasons for failure emerge. After a while the desire to have a baby can become a preoccupation, if not an obsession, as all thought and energy is focused on this. There is no doubt that the desire to reproduce is a very strong one, rooted in all sorts of often unrecognised needs. Part of this may be linked to a desire to reproduce something of ourselves, as a stake in the future. If reproductive technology takes us down a particular route, perhaps involving the use of donor sperm or eggs, without addressing issues like these, there may still remain a sense of failure in spite of successfully giving birth to a baby. In spite of the happiness this may bring, this grief may never be fully understood or resolved. Many fathers of children conceived by donor insemination still talk about their child's 'real' father.

Any assisted conception clinic providing treatment must also offer counselling before it is granted its licence. This counselling may be viewed as unnecessary by a couple if they see any need for it as a reflection of their ability to cope, rather than as a structured opportunity to discern some of the issues that the treatment can throw up. A skilled and sensitive counsellor can be extremely useful in raising some of the issues that need to be addressed, especially in cases of assisted conception. It is not just about making sure you understand the mechanics, and have 'come to terms' with problems with infertility. It is also about understanding what the implications of treatment might mean to you.

Although assisted conception may be the only option for some couples, and happily many babies have been successfully born because of it, in reality it is only essential for a few. If pregnancy does not seem to be happening, there is no reason to assume that this is the only option. Given the limitations of NHS resources (with each health authority defining its own criteria for treatment availability) which may be forced to exclude women over a certain age, and the costs of private treatment, it is also a limited option for many.

One of the purposes of this book is to outline the many ways in which women wanting to get pregnant can help themselves and their partner. And for every story of success through assisted conception, there is another of conception occurring against all odds. There is something in the nature of reproduction that defies all medical science, whether it is when babies do not happen or when, miraculously, they do. It could be loosely described as the spiritual component of babies, and the miracle of life. Whichever way you look at it, there are numerous stories of women who have conceived naturally after years of childlessness, after having adopted, after both successful and unsuccessful IVF treatment, and in their forties! While doctors are in the business of not raising expectations, and will only hazard a statistically-based guess at your chances, do take heart.

One woman, who had a completely blocked right tube while the left was a hydrosalpinx (a blockage with fluid and adhesions), and who had had a number of failed IVF treatments, had given up any idea of having a baby. She is a homeopath, and even though she was treating women with infertility problems, she considered herself more of a candidate for menopause treatment. At the age of forty-seven she found herself pregnant, and her perfectly healthy baby was born when she was forty-eight after an easy labour and delivery. What was difficult was everyone else's expectations of how her age was such a drawback but, after the results of the amniocentesis showed everything was fine, she stopped worrying and enjoyed her pregnancy.

If you are reading this book the chances are that you are either planning a pregnancy, or have been trying for several months without success so far. Although problems with infertility are covered, the primary focus of information is to provide you with all you need to know to help yourself most conclusively, whether this is about the timing of intercourse or when to seek medical help.

There are no easy answers, because what is right for one couple may not work for another. While one couple may feel that they want no medical intervention, another may want to take every step necessary to have a baby. And other couples decide first one thing, then change their minds. What is essential is access to the best information relevant to individual circumstance, and reading this book may be a first step or useful in providing additional information, depending on what is already known.

Having babies and raising a family is the most creative, stimulating, exhausting, rewarding, tedious, time-consuming, costly and exciting thing you will probably ever do. With so many contradictions further down the line, is it any wonder it can take some time to get going?

2 The Female fertility cycle

'Although I had a rough idea about my fertility cycle, what I knew was really only linked to having a period every four weeks or so. When it came to trying for a baby, I didn't really have a clear idea about when I ovulated. I guessed it was around the middle of my cycle, but until I started keeping some sort of record, I hadn't a clue how long this was!'

Clare, aged 27

'It wasn't until we'd been trying for a baby for six months that I realised how little I knew about how a baby was conceived, apart from the obvious details that is! I wish I'd found out a bit more about it before I started worrying, because once I knew about my own cycle it all seemed so straightforward and I got pregnant quite soon after that.'

Moyra, aged 34

While most women are aware that they have some sort of cycle of fertility, not everyone is clear about when they are most likely to get pregnant. Part of the reason for this is, perhaps, because we were told by our well-meaning elders that unprotected intercourse *always* ran the risk of pregnancy, in an attempt to promote carefulness about any sort of sexual contact. Even if our biology classes had been better than adequate, and we had read the leaflets that came free at the family planning clinic, a number of misconceptions about conception often remain.

Understanding the cycle of events that creates opportunities for conception is important, not only in attempting to achieve conception but also for understanding the reasons why conception is not always as straightforward as it might be. Certain events have to occur before pregnancy is fully established: ovulation; the meeting of the sperm and egg; fertilisation; implantation; and continuation of the pregnancy until the baby is born. Numerous things can go wrong at any of these stages and for those who find conception difficult, finding a solution cannot start until the reasons for this difficulty are identified. While we all have an idea, ranging from vague to explicit, about how our bodies function reproductively, it is always worth a recap. Just one small hitch at one stage of the procedure can mean the difference between success or failure. And if the problem is a combination of a number of factors, knowing where and how they occur makes it easier to assess the options available for finding a solution.

THE FERTILITY CYCLE

Every woman is born with a full complement of immature eggs in each of her ovaries and, during puberty, a fertility cycle controlled by hormones kicks in. Approximately every four weeks, one egg from one or other ovary begins to mature, ripen and is then shed. It is the availability of this egg that makes conception possible if it is fertilised by the male sperm and successfully implants in the womb.

The cycle of events that gives rise to ovulation is controlled by the secretion of hormones within a woman's body. Hormones are a sophisticated messenger system employed by the body to achieve a variety of functions, and are produced by a range of endocrine glands within the body, of which the ovaries are just two. Hormones are not just necessary for the purpose of fertility; there are other hormones like insulin, produced in the pancreas (an absence of which causes diabetes), that regulates the level of glucose in the blood. Hormones

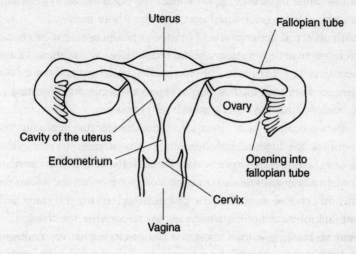

Female reproductive organs

secreted from one area of the body have an impact elsewhere, and the 'master' gland is the pituitary gland, located in the brain. The pituitary not only produces growth hormones, but chemicals that trigger other glands to produce their own hormones. For example, the thyroid gland is stimulated to produce hormones which regulate the body's metabolic rate – the speed at which energy is created and the body functions. And in a man, the pituitary gland stimulates the production of testosterone in the testes.

Without requiring a degree in endocrinology, it is useful to consider the complex and subtle interplay of hormones within the body when thinking about what impact this can have on a woman's fertility. It is the increase and decrease in levels of the four main hormones – follicle stimulating hormone (FSH), luteinising hormone (LH), oestrogen and progesterone that create the fertility cycle.

The two main female hormones of which most people are aware are oestrogen and progesterone. This is partly because these hormones do not just affect what is going on within the reproductive system, but also have a more generalised effect on the whole body.

At puberty, it is the effects of oestrogen production that cause the development of the secondary sexual characteristics of women. This is when a young girl begins to develop breasts, underarm and pubic hair begins to grow, body fat distribution begins to change and, eventually, she begins to have a regular menstrual period.

Oestrogen also has a direct effect on the internal reproduction organs, causing the lining of the womb to thicken and the end of the fallopian tube to move towards the ovarian follicle, and then contract in order to help any released ovum move down towards the womb. Its effect on cervical mucus is quite pronounced, making it thinner and more 'sperm-friendly'. Oestrogen is also responsible for changes in libido: its increase around mid-cycle can produce quite an increased sex-drive in some women. And its presence helps keep the skin supple and elastic. This elasticity also occurs in the skin folds of the vagina, making intercourse comfortable and giving birth possible.

On the down side, the changing impact of oestrogen during their cycle can cause fluid retention in some women, as it encourages the body's cells to retain salt. This can make breasts uncomfortable, and give rise to feelings of 'bloatedness' in susceptible women. But not all women react in this way, and not all react in this way every month. The other very important function of oestrogen is that it helps keep bones strong by facilitating the uptake of calcium necessary to their density. And there is strong evidence to show that, up to menopause, women are protected in part against coronary heart disease by the presence of oestrogen. So overall, its advantages are plain to see!

Progesterone is mainly responsible for preparing a woman's body for pregnancy, which it will attempt to do following ovulation. One of the effects of progesterone is also to prepare the breasts, which can swell slightly prior to a period. In addition, progesterone, unlike oestrogen, has a diuretic effect – salt is lost from the body and, as a result, fluid.

With all this internal activity, it becomes clear how very responsive women's bodies are to the changing hormonal levels and the effects this can have on them generally. It is also part of what makes a woman so very individual: although the basic equipment might be the same, what influences it is susceptible to infinite variety. So for each woman who interprets her mood as irritable before her period, there may be another who experiences this as a time of increased introspection and greater creativity. And for every woman who dislikes the feeling of tension in her breasts mid-cycle, there will be another who finds it makes her feel particularly sexy.

'I had a terrible time in my teens with fluid retention before a period. It made me feel extremely uncomfortable and, because my periods were very irregular, I was never sure when I would be affected. Then, after going on the pill in my twenties for a few years, things seemed to settle down. Now, after having had a baby, it's not a problem.'

Tracey, aged 29

'I always know when my period's due because I can never park the car in one easy go! But the rest of the time, I'm an excellent driver.'

Angela, aged 37

'I'm a freelance graphic designer, and I find the time just before I ovulate is when I'm most effective. Then work just zips along. But the week before a period, I really have to push myself. I've just learnt to bear this in mind when I'm planning my workload.'

Sheena, aged 33

'I always get quite a specific low-backache the day before my period is due. It's very accurate, and quite a useful reminder really!'

Lizzie, aged 22

By the same token, women will find that their ability to become pregnant differs – even within the same family. While one woman may conceive with apparent ease, her sister may have a quite different experience. So although it is always useful to compare notes and discuss things with other women, always bear in mind that you are totally individual and what is worth thinking about is how *you* work; get to know your own fertility cycle.

This cycle actually begins in an area of the brain called the hypothalamus. Here, a hormone called gonadotrophin releasing hormone (GnRH) stimulates the pituitary gland to release the hormone FSH into the bloodstream. This stimulates the development of a number of follicles in the ovary, in which the eggs are housed, with one becoming dominant. Very occasionally more than one continues to develop and, if hormone treatment is being given in preparation for IVF, for example, then several follicles will continue to develop. However, under normal circumstances the dominant follicle secretes greater and greater amounts of oestrogen. The rising level of oestrogen in the blood has three effects:

- it inhibits the continued production of FSH, so reducing the possibility of more than one egg being released;
- the glands in the cervix are stimulated to produce mucus that is much 'wetter', enabling sperm to journey more effectively up the female reproductive tract to a possible egg;
- the lining of the womb begins to thicken, in preparation for possible implantation of a fertilised egg and pregnancy.

The ever-increasing amount of oestrogen from the maturing follicle in turn stimulates the production of LH, from the pituitary gland, which is effective in making the follicle rupture and shed its ripened egg. This is ovulation.

After ovulation, the empty follicle – now called the corpus luteum – starts secreting progesterone. Progesterone is a hormone which, like oestrogen, has a number of effects. In this instance, it prevents the pituitary gland from secreting any more FSH or LH, so preventing any further ovulation in that cycle. Progesterone also makes cervical mucus much thicker and stickier, and it forms something of a plug at the cervix. If the egg is not fertilised, the corpus luteum responsible for

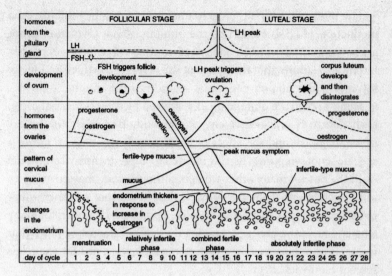

Fluctuating hormone levels over a complete cycle, and their effect

progesterone secretion degenerates and stops production. This process always takes fourteen days from ovulation – it is the only fixed time interval in the whole cycle. Then, without the presence of progesterone in the blood, the thickened lining of the womb literally comes away in a small flow of blood creating what we know as a period. This complete drop in all hormonal levels is what is necessary to kick-start the whole procedure into action again. However, if a fertilised egg does implant in the womb and pregnancy occurs, then the corpus luteum continues to secrete progesterone until the placenta is mature enough to take over its production at around three months.

How the contraceptive pill works

Combined hormonal contraceptive pills work by simulating the effect of one hormone over another, based on the principle that if the body can be fooled into thinking it has ovulated, then it will not produce an egg and so the cycle of fertility is inhibited.

The mini-pill, which is progesterone only, works by inhibiting the production of FSH and LH by the pituitary gland. Ovulation is not always prevented so, as an additional contraceptive measure, progesterone also ensures that the mucus at the cervix is too thick and sticky to prevent the smooth passage of sperm into the womb.

Some women are quite markedly affected by their hormonal cycle, both positively and negatively, as previously discussed. At the extreme, negative end the effect of female sex hormones can create a specific set of symptoms, usually referred to as pre-menstrual syndrome or PMS. But for many other women, although they may be aware of mild fluctuations in mood, hunger, fluid retention, or other symptoms, these are not so great as to cause a problem. However, for many women one of the benefits of taking the oral contraceptive pill is that it somehow re-balances their own hormonal cycles, making them less susceptible to its effects.

The two phases of the fertility cycle

Another important point to consider with the fertility cycle is that it has two distinct phases, but only one fixed time interval as previously mentioned: this is the fourteen days between ovulation and a period, if conception has not occurred. This is an important point to grasp when you are trying to work out *when* in your cycle your ovulate because it all depends on the length of your cycle. You will only ovulate fourteen days *after* the first day of your period if your cycle is an exact twenty-eight days long, because this will also be fourteen days *before* your period was due.

The first phase, up to ovulation, is described as the follicular phase and this can be of variable length. Then the fourteen-day phase between ovulation and leading up to menstruation is called the luteal phase because of the activity of the corpus luteum. For example, if your normal average cycle is thirty days long, then you are probably ovulating on around day sixteen of your cycle. If your cycle varies from one occasion to another, then working out when you ovulate can only be done retrospectively, unless you use other indicators of ovulation which are specific to you.

However, if you are as regular as clockwork, even if your normal cycle is only twenty-five days long, then you are probably ovulating at around day eleven of your cycle. Understanding about when in your cycle you are most likely to be ovulating is crucial because if, as with the above cycle, you were planning intercourse in the hope of conceiving on day fourteen of your cycle, then ovulation would have already occurred. Likewise, with a very long cycle of say thirty-six days, ovulation is probably occurring at around day twenty-two – quite a big difference from day fourteen!

This is why, when you are trying to conceive a baby, it is worth spending a little time understanding the fertility cycle and, in particular, your own. There are also other indicators of fertility which are worth considering and these have been the subject of extensive research and investigation, in order to pinpoint ovulation, as far as is possible, in order to *avoid* conception: natural family planning. And this information is extremely valuable in helping to achieve conception. In fact, about 40% of those who consult trained Natural Family Planning (NFP) teachers do so in order to achieve pregnancy. Certainly having the benefit of someone who can explain, in person, your own fertility cycle and its indicators and also provide the support and counselling necessary, which is what a trained NFP teacher can do, is beneficial. Not only is it helpful to work towards achieving pregnancy naturally, it is also very reassuring to see that ovulation is occurring and consequently feel confident that conception is possible. Contact Fertility UK or the National Family Planning Teachers' Association (see Useful Addresses) for further information.

INDICATORS OF FERTILITY

The two main indicators of fertility are a change of body temperature, and a change in cervical mucus. There is a slight, but definite increase

Ovulation occurs approximately 14 days *before* a
period, regardless of the length of a woman's cycle

Long cycle

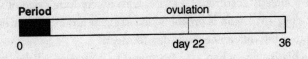

Period   ovulation

0   day 22   36

Average cycle

Period   ovulation

0   day 14   28

Short cycle

Period   ovulation

0   day 11   25

Diagram demonstrating different lengths of the two phases of the fertility cycle for average cycles of 25, 28 and 36 days in basal body temperature (BBT) after ovulation because of the effect of the progesterone secreted by the corpus luteum, after the egg has been shed. Basal body temperature is the temperature of the body at rest, without any influence from activity, eating or drinking. Because the temperature shift after ovulation is definite, but slight – only a couple of points of a degree – this is important. However, the BBT continues at this slightly elevated rate for the rest of the cycle.

Temperature changes

What charting your temperature over a couple of cycles may show you is a) whether or not you are ovulating, and b) if you are, whereabouts in your cycle this is occurring. What it *will not* tell you is when you are about to ovulate, although some women report a slight drop in their BBT the day before it increases on ovulation. However, many women still find it invaluable because it helps in their understanding of their own, individual fertility. While remembering to take your temperature every morning, before getting up, can be tedious it still might be worth considering for a number of months in order to reassure you that your other, individual, indicators of fertility are accurate.

The most useful tip to remember about temperature charting is to try and take it at roughly the same time each day and if, for example, you've overslept one morning, to make a note of this on the chart. You can then be sure whether any unexpected variation that shows up is specific to this – or to any other reason; perhaps to having a slight hangover, or a cold, which could influence your body temperature slightly.

A digital thermometer is particularly useful if you are not confident about using a mercury thermometer, although it is possible to buy these calibrated more clearly for easier use. Taking your temperature by mouth is much more accurate than underarm, and you need to leave the thermometer in place for at least a minute. You must also have nothing to drink – either hot or cold – immediately beforehand. If you are uncertain about any aspect of taking your temperature,

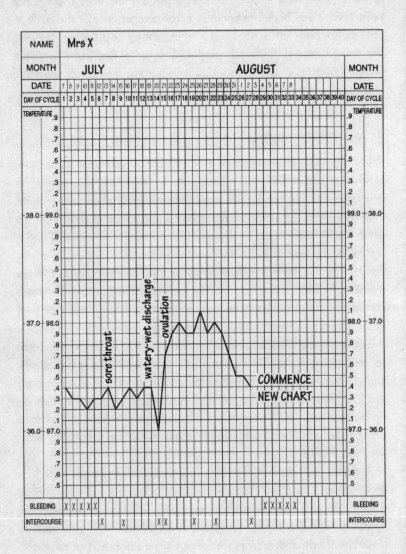

Temperature chart

then your best port of call for advice is, again, Fertility UK. Not only can they advise you, they can also give you the name of a local teacher to contact for help, and provide you with both thermometers and specially-designed charts. These make the information much more visually accessible, and they do mean it is much easier to see exactly what is going on.

Mucus secretions

For many women, the best indicator of their approaching ovulation is the changing pattern of cervical mucus secretion. Even without paying much attention to their bodies, most women are aware that they produce more cervical mucus some times than at others. Advertisements for panty liners and other sanitary protection products are acknowledging this when they describe those 'in between days' when, apparently, we need some added protection.

The cervix, as described above, has surface cells that produce mucus. This keeps the vagina lubricated and comfortable and also has a role to play in the transportation of sperm. Mucus is produced in response to the increase in oestrogen that is produced up to ovulation. Not only do the cervical cells produce more mucus, it is also quite specifically more copious, watery, thinner, clear and 'stretchier' in consistency, leading up to ovulation.

Immediately following a period, little or no cervical mucus is produced. Any in evidence is likely to be thick and opaque. While a woman might be aware of some one day, there may be none at all the next. However, as the cycle progresses, for most women this situation changes quite noticeably. Again, it may require observation over a number of cycles before a woman can feel confident that cervical mucus is a relevant indicator of her fertility. But because the change from what is referred to as 'fertile-type' mucus (clear, watery, stretchy) back to 'infertile type' (tacky, scant, opaque) and back again can be quite dramatic, and because it marks the approach of ovulation so clearly, many women find it very useful. Once ovulation has occurred, mucus secretion influenced by the reduction in oestrogen and increase in progesterone, changes within several hours.

Fertile-type mucus is sometimes described as being very much like raw egg white, and one of its roles is to transport sperm through the female reproductive tract to a waiting egg. The natural acidity of the vagina, which is detrimental to sperm, is neutralised by the cervical mucus produced around ovulation. So being aware of cervical mucus as a sign of approaching ovulation, and timing intercourse to maximise on this, also has the benefit of additionally favourable conditions for conception. Given that ovulation occurs within forty-eight hours of maximum mucus secretions, and sperm can live for between two and five days in a favourable environment, it becomes possible to work out the most favourable times for conception with this knowledge. In a World Health Organisation study, it was found that 97% of women could accurately interpret their mucus symptoms after only three months.

The production of cervical mucus can be affected by some drugs for colds and sinusitis – those that are designed to reduce mucus secretion in the nose can also affect the cervix. In addition, a vaginal infection that produces a discharge can affect the quality of mucus secretions. This is more of a problem for women who are not familiar with their own mucus pattern. Those who are can generally tell the difference.

Another effect of the fluctuating hormones of the fertility cycle is on the cervix itself, and not just on its ability to produce different types of mucus. As ovulation approaches, the cervix softens and the cervical os (opening) releases slightly, while the cervix moves back from the vagina, making it less immediately accessible. This is in contrast to the position and feel of the cervix during the rest of the cycle.

Changes in the cervix

Becoming familiar with your cervix, and what it feels like, can be another way of assessing your fertility and the most fertile phase of your cycle. What it requires, however, is monitoring of changes to the cervix over one, if not more, cycles to become familiar with them. Accessing your cervix takes a little practice and it is best to find a way that is comfortable for you, and stick to that position each time. That way, any detectable change has nothing to do with a change in your body position. It is also perfectly hygienic if you wash your hands beforehand. Once you have found your cervix, it is distinguishable from the interior walls of the vagina because it is quite firm and definite in comparison to these. One comparison made suggested that the cervix was similar, in feeling, to the tip of the nose. While the cervical os may only be recognisable as a slight indentation in women who have not had children, in those who have had children it is much more obvious. However, even trained gynaecologists can occasionally have difficulty reaching the cervix in a patient, and actually appreciating the subtle changes in the cervix which vary according to the menstrual cycle can be a difficult technique to master for oneself, so do not worry if you are unable to do this.

Other signs and symptoms of ovulation may be more subtle, but for some women can be very distinctive. Because it is not only our sex organs that are responsive to the fluctuation in hormones, we may notice a change in skin texture for example, or an increased yearning for carbohydrates. Many women also find that their rising hormone levels over a cycle affect their libido and make them feel sexier and, conversely, later in their cycle they may experience the reverse.

Mid-cycle pain

Some women find that around the time of actual ovulation they experience either a quite sharp, one-sided abdominal pain or perhaps a generalised gripey-ness. Unless on the look-out for minor signs like these, it is easy to miss or confuse them. It is only over a number of cycles that it becomes possible to be sure that a particular sign or symptom is linked to ovulation.

Checklist of main indicators:

- ◆ temperature changes;
- ◆ changes in cervical mucus secretion;
- ◆ accessibility and feel of cervix;
- ◆ mid-cycle pain or 'mittelschmerz'.

It becomes increasingly easy to identify a variety of signs and symptoms that indicate approaching ovulation if they are being considered in the light of other indicators. Combining these indicators, in order to become more aware of the rhythms and changes that occur within an individual fertility cycle, is especially helpful when trying to assess opportunities for conception.

'It took me a while to get the hang of taking my temperature – and interpreting it – accurately, but what was dramatic was the difference in my cervical mucus secretions just prior to ovulation. Now I don't bother to take my temperature, but I know when I'm going to ovulate and I have a right-sided pain at that time too. I've conceived both my babies knowing when I was ovulating.'

Amrit, aged 37

'I had been using fertility awareness as a form of contraception in between all my babies. I have five – all planned!'

Sally, aged 40

'It wasn't until I had been charting for a while, that I was able to see that I really was ovulating – thanks to the help of my NFP teacher. I think it was this that gave me the confidence to relax, and believe it was possible for me to conceive. Anyway, after nine years of trying, I got pregnant.'

Monica, aged 33

It is also important to be aware of external influences to fertility indicators. Numerous things can influence something as finely-tuned as the female cycle. A woman may already be aware of how she is influenced when she notices fluctuations in, say, the length of her normal cycle. But for a woman who is charting her temperature over the course of her cycle, getting any infection that gives her a temperature will affect her readings. Anything that affects our circadian rhythms, shift work or jet lag, for example, can have an impact. Even a stressful period of work, with deadlines and long hours, can influence a cycle. It will not necessarily reduce fertility but can affect the length of a cycle and the timing of ovulation.

Numerous drugs, not including the contraceptive pill, can cause irregularities in a menstrual cycle. These include some tranquillisers, so check with your doctor. In addition, medicines used to treat migraine, nausea or vomiting, and those for travel sickness, need to be checked. Any drug that causes an increase in the level of prolactin, which can delay or suppress ovulation, needs to be avoided when trying to conceive.

Any preparations containing cortisone, commonly used in the treatment of asthma, hay fever and rheumatic problems may need to be considered. Cortisone is an adrenal hormone, and prolonged use may have an effect on the fertility cycle, perhaps causing irregularities. While these are quite specific instances of medication, relevant to their possible impact on the fertility cycle, it is also wise to consider all forms of medication and their general impact. This is covered more fully in chapter 4, Fit to conceive? It is important to note that anyone taking corticosteroids should always consult their doctor if they are considering stopping medication.

Ovulation predictor kits can be helpful for some women. These are a commercially manufactured home urine test, available from chemists and pharmacies. They contained five specially prepared urine dip-sticks, sensitive to the presence of luteinising hormone (LH) in the urine. A surge in LH occurs just prior to ovulation so, once this has been detected, you are likely to ovulate within the next two to three days. Timing intercourse for this time can help improve the chances for conception.

These kits are not cheap, but can be very reassuring, showing a woman that interpretation of her own self-assessed indicators of fertility, and approaching ovulation, are correct. Full instructions are given in each pack, plus some useful additional information about fertility and conception.

3 Male fertility

A man's general health is just as important to conception as a woman's, although this often gets overlooked by fertility experts, who tend to be gynaecologists and obstetricians, specialists in female, not male, reproductive health. Problems in conception are often thought to be wholly the woman's, but this is not the case. When a couple have a problem with conception, the problem is only with the woman in around 35–40% of the time, with the man between 30–35% of the time, and results from a combined problem for the rest.

Unlike women, who are born with a full complement of eggs in their ovaries, from puberty men are constantly producing sperm. Within the man's scrotum are the testes, inside which sperm are produced. Initially immature spermatids are produced in the rete testis which precedes the epididymis. The development continues as it journeys through approximately forty feet of the epididymis, which takes between two to three weeks. It is here that the sperm mature, and become capable of motility and fertilisation, over this period of time. An estimated 4–5 million spermatozoa are produced, per gram of testicle, per day. From here the vas deferens transport the sperm at ejaculation, mixed with secretions from the seminal vesicles and the prostate gland, via the urethra to the penis. These secretions are important for both nurturing the sperm, and for facilitating the transportation process.

Through an understanding of the way sperm is produced, the fact that it is produced so continuously and is consequently more easily

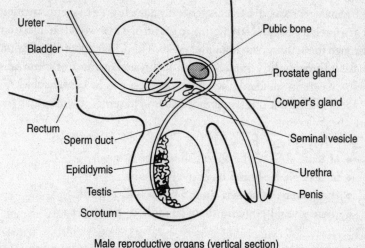

Ureter
Bladder
Rectum
Sperm duct
Epididymis
Testis
Scrotum
Pubic bone
Prostate gland
Cowper's gland
Seminal vesicle
Urethra
Penis

Male reproductive organs (vertical section)

Cross section of male testes, scrotum, urethra and penis

influenced by a man's health and surroundings, and the extraordinary journey it makes prior to ejaculation, makes it possible to see how and why problems can occur. The internal diameter of the epididymis is so fine that any external damage can have a big impact on its internal workings. A varicose vein in the testicle, although it is causing no pain, may be just enough to create a blockage. While ejaculation produces seminal fluid, only microscopic examination can tell the real story.

The fact that the testes are outside the body, and at a cooler body temperature, suggests that over-heating in this area, perhaps by wearing tight pants and trousers, can be detrimental to sperm production. Certainly if sperm production is low, then this may be worth a thought, but taking cold baths and splashing the testicles with icy-cold water probably will not achieve much; there was not a notable drop in male fertility when fashion decreed skin-tight jeans.

At ejaculation the volume of semen should be between two and five ml. and contain over 20 million sperm per ml. This apparently enormous quantity is produced for important reasons. First, only a proportion of sperm produced are normal, active and able to fertilise an egg. Second, the female reproductive tract is generally quite hostile to sperm, treating it as a foreign body and attempting to get rid of it as it would an infection through the activity of its immune system. Third, only about 5% of sperm make it through the cervix. So if the quality and quantity of sperm falls below a certain standard, the knock-on effect can be considerable.

Generally, what one would hope to find in terms of semen analysis are the following:

◆ at least 40% of the sperm should be normal;
◆ at least 40% should be actively moving;
◆ the volume of semen should be around 2–5 ml;
◆ there should be more than 20 million sperm per ml.

The production of sperm, because it happens so continuously, can be influenced by a variety of factors, which is why general good health in a man is important when trying to conceive, covered more fully in the following chapter, Fit to conceive? Smoking and alcohol can have a negative effect on sperm production, which may or may not matter depending on how good production was already. Marijuana is well-documented as reducing sperm production. That said, it is also well-known that well into their seventies men are quite capable of producing sperm and impregnating a woman.

REDUCTION IN SPERM COUNTS

There's no doubt that sperm counts have diminished, from around 87 million sperm per millilitre in 1989 to 62 million sperm per millilitre in 2002, which is a significant drop of almost a third, 29%. Previous research has recorded sperm counts falling around the world by an estimated 50% in the past fifty years, but scientists have not yet established the full extent of external influences that may affect a decline in the quantity and quality of sperm. Drug use, alcohol, smoking and obesity are among the factors most frequently blamed. The effects of the environment, including the presence of pesticides, chemicals and radioactive material, have also been linked to decreases in sperm production and fertility.

ASSESSING A MAN'S FERTILITY

Semen analysis provides such a valuable look at the male contribution to conception, and at specific problems, because it can immediately identify those steps that can be taken to improve the quality and quantity of sperm production. In addition, if there is a specific problem that can indicate a physical, or genetic, problem then further tests can be decided upon.

A man's normal fertility can fluctuate, and is always a matter of degree. So if there is a degree of sub-fertility, where the sperm count is borderline, for example, the reassuring news is that it can usually be improved. It's also important to remember that fertility is not the same as virility – an infertile man can continue to be extremely virile, for example after a vasectomy! Identifying whether there is a problem, and to what degree, enables couples to define what their parameters of fertility are, and work with that information whether it means major lifestyle changes, or exploring assisted conception.

DNA FRAGMENTATION

Advances in semen analysis means that not only can the quantity and quality of sperm be assessed, but also its genetic material. Genetic abnormalities in an embryo are one of the major causes of early miscarriage, as this prevents normal development and the embryo dies. While this was previously thought to be a fault with the woman's egg, or a random mutation, it's now becoming increasingly evident that chromosomal abnormalities in sperm – which can now be screened for – can be a major contributing factor to infertility. While genetic abnormalities can be inherited, they can also be caused by environmental pollutants, and lifestyle factors including caffeine, alcohol and smoking. Sperm are particularly vulnerable to this because they are in constant production, but the good news is that relevant changes have a big and positive impact.

Standard sperm testing doesn't yet include checking for DNA fragmentation, for example, as routine. DNA is the genetic material within the chromosomes of the sperm cells. If there are errors in this material or damage to it, for example in the structural arrangement of the cells, this can make conception impossible. The flawed sperm can't produce a normally fertilised egg, resulting either in early miscarriage or 'unexplained' infertility.

In a normally fertile man, between 2% and 13% of sperm are genetically abnormal. Age has an impact on the amount of genetically abnormal material carried by sperm, while research has shown that caffeine, alcohol, cigarette smoking and exposure to environmental pollution significantly increase the percentage of abnormality. There is also a normal amount of DNA fragmentation in sperm, where an element of breakage in the DNA strands occurs. Under normal circumstances, the woman's egg has a capacity to repair low-level fragmentation at fertilisation, but if the level reaches a certain threshold, this is no longer possible resulting in an abnormal conception and early miscarriage.

Standard tests don't usually cover DNA fragmentation, but it is worth requesting this because sperm DNA fragmentation is known to compromise male fertility. Men who have had recent infections, like the flu, or any form of genito-urinary infection should have this checked. Studies have shown that antibiotic treatment for residual infections can help reduce DNA fragmentation rates, and reducing oxidative stress also showed good results, according to one study published in 2005 by the American Society of Andrology. Here, a gram a day each of orial antioxidants vitamin C and E was given over a two month period and showed improved results.

Having sex more often, at least daily, will also reduce the risk of DNA damage, according to research carried out by Dr David Greening from the Sydney IVF treatment centre in Wollongong, New South Wales.

While it was not entirely clear why this helped, it is thought that daily sex reduces exposure to harmful molecules in the testicular ducts. Participants in the study, who already had higher than normal DNA sperm damage, were asked to ejaculate daily for seven days without making any other lifestyle changes. Sperm damage fell by an average of 10 percent, plus the aibility of the sperm to reach a viable egg also rose, even while volume of semen and concentration of sperm fell slightly.

AGE

Although age is considered less of a problem with regard to male fertility than it is in a woman, there is a change in the quality and production of sperm as men age. The leydig cells, that produce testosterone, decrease in number over time so the secretion of this hormone is reduced. The resulting decrease in sperm count and motility, and an increase in the numbers of abnormal sperm, is part of the effect of diminished hormonal output. There is also an increase in chromosomal abnormalities in the sperm of older men, which, if they result in conception can lead to birth defects.

A recent study showed that men, aged thirty-five or older, are 50% less likely, over a twelve-month period, to achieve a conception with a fertile female partner than are men who are younger. This decline in fertility is thought to be attributable to the 'male menopause' when levels of male hormones decrease.

A word, however, on the use of Viagra, the use of which could contribute to fertility problems. Dr David Glenn, a consultant gynaecologist at Queen's University Belfast, has found that Viagra can damage the acrosome in the sperm, needed to break down the enzymes surrounding the egg that allow penetration, without which fertilisation can't occur. Concern was raised when it was found that some IVF clinics were prescribing Viagra to men to help boost fertility results. If you are using Viagra while also trying to get our partner pregnant, you may need to discuss this with your doctor.

4 Fit to conceive?

'I felt really fit and healthy before I got pregnant and I think it helped a lot when I had bad morning sickness during the first three months. I actually lost weight initially, but once I stopped feeling sick I was fine, and felt terrific throughout the rest of the time.'

Sheena, aged 33

'I have insulin-dependent diabetes, so I was pretty nervous about what effect being pregnant would have. Thankfully I got a lot of support from the pre-conception clinic attached to my local diabetes unit, and that helped. I conceived fairly easily, and Daniel was born at term – a straightforward delivery – perfectly healthy and we had no problems.'

Dawn, aged 27

It goes without saying that looking after yourself, and being sensible about your health, is a useful preliminary to having a baby. However, there are a number of misconceptions that need to be addressed. Even the strongest, fittest men can have a low sperm count. Women who live a healthy life can still have a hormonal imbalance, while the fact that babies are born to women with drug habits shows that even the least healthy among us are still capable of conception. It may hardly seem fair, but fertility has little respect for personal circumstance one way or another.

That said, there are occasions when the steps you take to increase your general health and well-being are extremely sensible not only for conception but, should you conceive a baby, then for the benefit of your continuing health during pregnancy and after the birth. Babies are wonderfully efficient at taking what they need from you for their growth and development in the womb, so it is likely to be the mother, rather than her baby, who takes the toll for this if her general health is below par. And, because the first few months of a baby's life are so physically and emotionally draining for the parents, it is preferable to be as fit and healthy as possible before you start.

It is also essential to keep some sense of perspective about any problems with conceiving that you may be facing. Focusing obsessionally on what you eat and drink prior to conception places unnaturally high expectations on yourself, when a more relaxed attitude would be more helpful. The aim of this chapter is to not only look at some general information about health and fitness, but also to look at some of those health issues specific to conception and pregnancy, while debunking some of the myths that prevail.

NUTRITION

Before thinking about what you put into the body, it's worth thinking about what your body does with it once it arrives there. Nutrition isn't just about choosing good food, it's about eating in a way that allows the body to make the best of it. Too many of us eat in a hurry, while feeling tense, or late at night – which makes it difficult for our digestive system to work adequately. So nutrition isn't just about what you eat, but how you eat. For example, the average length of time it takes an American to eat a Big Mac is eleven minutes; the average length of time it takes for a French person is twenty-two minutes. Without advocating eating a Big Mac, it says something for two different approaches to food – and the consequences: the French seem able to eat without getting fat, and maybe the rate at which they eat has something to do with it. Eating in a relaxed way enables your digestive system to get the most out of the food you eat.

The digestive tract is the largest endocrine gland in the body. Digestion begins in the mouth when you chew and with the release of salivary juices, and the enzyme ptyalin or salivary amylaze, which starts the conversion of cooked starches to maltose. The stomach, only the size of a fist, receives the chewed food where it is mixed with more digestive juices, including the enzymes pepsin and rennin, and one called the intrinsic factor that is necessary for the absorption of the anti-anaemia factor. Without the secretion of these enzymes, the digestive system can't work properly and the first stage of secretion begins before food actually reaches the stomach, stimulated by the sight, smell and chewing of food. Eating should be a multi-sensorial process in order for digestion to work best! Take time for your meals, and enjoy them, as you will digest your food much more productively.

From the stomach, the liquefied food, or chyme, moves into the duodenum, where further enzymes slow its process, allowing time for the addition of other digestive factors. The journey of the food eaten onward through the small intestine helps complete the conversion of proteins to amino-acids, maltose (carbohydrates) to monosaccharides, and fats are emulsified by bile from the gall bladder and converted to fatty acids and glycerol. Only in these converted forms can these be used effectively by the body. Anything that interferes with this process, for example poor secretion of digestive juices if meals are eaten in great haste or late at night, or when you are stressed and anxious, can affect the level of benefit you get from the food you eat.

The small intestine is also crucially important for the immune system. 80% of immune cells are made here, so the function of the small intestine is integral to a strong immune system. The small intestine is lined with thousands of small finger-like projections, called villi, where the liquefied food we have eaten comes into extremely close proximity to blood capillaries and the absorption of nutrients takes place. If food passes through the small intestine too quickly, or there is any sort of tension or spasm that reduces the blood supply to this area during this crucial process, then the absorption of nutrients is inhibited.

The large intestine is mostly concerned with the re-absorption of liquid, and the elimination of the bulky waste products and by-products of digestion. When this elimination is regular and effective, helped by an adequate intake of dietary fibre and water, and not hindered by bowel problems like a candida infection or irritable bowel syndrome, then the body isn't burdened by toxins, which result from an accumulation of waste products in the bowel, and digestive and general health is good.

DIET

There is no doubt that the nutritional value of what we eat is important and that a balanced diet low in saturated fats, high in fibre, and with lots of fresh vegetables and fruit is beneficial to your general health at all times. As a nation we do tend to eat too much in the way of processed foods, and too much sugar content in one form or another. Current dietary advice makes the following recommendations:

Fruit and vegetables

Five servings per day, including at least one green leafy vegetable.

A serving is the equivalent of a piece of fruit (apple, orange or banana, etc.); about 4 oz (110g) of vegetables; a small glass of fruit juice, for example.

Bread, potatoes, rice and other cereals

Four to five servings a day.

A serving is the equivalent of a slice of bread; a 1-1.5 oz (30-45g) bowl of breakfast cereal; 5-6.5 oz (140-180g) of potatoes, yams or sweet potatoes; 5-7.5 oz (140-220g) of cooked rice or pasta; a roll or chapatti, for example.

Milk and dairy products

Three servings a day.

A serving is the equivalent of a third of a pint of milk (0.2 litre/ 200 ml); 1 oz (30g) of cheese; a small carton of yoghurt, for example.

Meat, fish and other sources of protein including vegetable pulses

Two servings a day.

A serving is the equivalent of 4.5 oz (130g) of beef, lamb, pork, tinned tuna or white fish; 3 oz (85g) of poultry or oily fish; 3.5-5 oz (100-140g) of vegetable pulses (kidney beans, lentils, black-eyed beans, baked beans, etc); 1 oz (30g) of nuts, for example.

If you follow this brief outline it should ensure that you get a good balance of protein and carbohydrate, providing you with the nutrients, vitamins and minerals, and fibre you need. Further information on the most up-to-date recommendations can be obtained from www.nhs.uk/Planners/pregnancycareplanner/pages/Eating.aspx.

There are other general recommendations about reducing the amount of highly processed foods you eat if they usually form part of your diet. This is partly because they are notoriously low in fibre and high in hidden fats and sugars, but also because their nutritional content is reduced through the processing. Opting for wholefoods, whether this means substituting granary bread for white, eating wholewheat pastas and brown rice, or increasing your intake of fresh vegetables and fruit, automatically helps your nutritional status.

Reducing the fat content of our diets continues to be an important contribution to general health. Changing to skimmed milk instead of full-fat, grilling food rather than frying it, using low-fat spreads instead of butter, are all now familiar guidelines and worth adhering to. If this means making rather more of a change in your diet and lifestyle than you had anticipated, remember that it is not just beneficial for you and your partner, and potentially your unborn child, you will also be introducing good dietary principles that will influence the continuing health of your child for all of his or her life.

'I couldn't bear the taste of skimmed milk at first, so had to use semi-skimmed. Now I don't like the taste of full-fat milk at all!'

Tracey, aged 29

'I had got into very bad eating habits. I worked long hours so tended to miss breakfast, grab a sandwich for lunch, and then eat out in the evening. I had to make a conscious effort at first just to take ten minutes for a bowl of muesli in the morning, and not rely on a cup of black coffee. I also made a conscious effort to prepare food at home in the evenings, inviting people round instead of going out. I definitely feel much better for it overall.'

Judith, aged 31

'I knew I had to lose a bit of weight before I got pregnant, but I also knew it wasn't the best time to try a drastic diet. So I just changed various key things, according to a booklet I got from the Health Education Authority. Over time it was enough to make quite a difference. Combined with walking to work, instead of taking the bus, as often as I could, I lost half a stone in six months without trying and feel much better for it. And I'm now six months pregnant.'

Tricia, aged 35

Whether or not you choose organically produced fruit and vegetables is up to you: there is no conclusive evidence that it is more beneficial when trying to get pregnant. Availability and cost – unless you are fortunate to grow your own or live near an organic supplier – can make this difficult, although many supermarkets now stock a range of organic fruit and vegetables. Certainly there may be some sense in choosing those vegetables which you might eat raw, like carrots, if you are concerned about the use of pesticides. With fruit, you can always peel an apple or pear if you are not convinced that washing is enough.

The same goes for organically produced meat: cost and availability are also likely to be considerations. With meat, unless you are a vegetarian, it would be better for you nutritionally to eat it, organic or not, to ensure an adequate iron intake. While iron is available through other dietary sources, it is most directly available in meat. A proportion of women, estimated to be around 20%, are sub-clinically anaemic. That is, they show no gross signs of anaemia and are functioning adequately although on a low haemoglobin level. While this is not specifically detrimental to your health, or even to your chances of conceiving, and easily rectified with a more balanced diet, it may contribute to feeling rather tired and run down occasionally. Certainly haemoglobin levels are something that is checked in early pregnancy, and although iron supplements are now no longer routinely given, many women still benefit from an increased iron intake during pregnancy.

THE BENEFITS OF FULL FAT DAIRY

New research from the exhaustive, longitudinal *Nurses' Health Study* (which was started in 1976 and expanded in 1989) that has scrutinised the lives of nearly 116,000 women, provided some interesting new evidence on fertility, covered by Drs Jorge Chavarro and Walter Willett in their 2008 book *The Fertility Diet*.

The study involved more than 18,000 women aged 24 to 42 who had no history of infertility and had tried to become pregnant between 1991 and 1999. Researchers found that the women who drank whole milk and ate full-fat dairy products were more fertile than those who stuck to low-fat products. This could help explain the apparent increase in infertility in the West as fashion-conscious young women try to eat healthily and stay slim by shunning full-fat dairy products. It seemed that eating two or more servings of low-fat dairy products a day – which could include a portion of cottage cheese and a low-fat yoghurt –

increased the risk of failed ovulation by 85 per cent, researchers found. But women who ate at least one serving of high-fat dairy food a day cut their risk of infertility from this cause by 27 per cent.

Full-fat ice cream was suddenly on the fertility menu! The more ice cream the women ate the lower their risk of infertility. Women eating ice cream two or more times a week had a 38 per cent lower risk of infertility than those who consumed ice cream less than once a week. Including full-fat dairy in an otherwise balanced diet, coupled with adequate exercise, may just tip the balance in women who have otherwise unexplained ovulatory problems.

ACID/ALKALINE BALANCE

For the body to function properly, its basic state needs to be alkaline, and this is crucial for fertility. The increased female cervical secretions around the time of ovulation need to be alkaline to protect the sperm from the normally acid environment of the vagina. Production of sperm requires an alkaline environment. The acid/alkaline balance needs to be 20/80 for optimum functioning, but our typical Westernised diet creates an acid/alkaline imbalance.

To get your body back in balance, and enhance fertility, it is essential to get back to an alkaline state. We all eat far too many acidic foods. Our diet is generally too high in protein and too low in carbohydrate. Weight loss diets based on this ratio are catastrophically bad for both men and women when it comes to trying to get pregnant.

The acid/alkaline balance is measured by what is called the pH level. The pH scale is between 1 and 14, with any measurement below 7 indicating acidity. The 'normal' pH level that is considered healthy is 7.4, but is often below this in adults because of their diet and lifestyle. Each calibration on the pH scale is 10 times the previous one so, for example, if your pH level is 6.4 rather than 7.4, it is 10 times more acidic. Many adults have a pH reading – from saliva, urine, or blood – of below the pH norm. For good health, and this includes avoiding other health problems like arthritis, heart disease, osteoporosis, cancer (cancer cells find it hard to exist in an alkaline environment) and kidney disease, keeping the body in an alkaline state is beneficial.

Acid/alkaline balance is easier to maintain than it is to correct, so it's well worth thinking about the dietary changes that need to be made in the long term, as well as in the short term. Keeping the range of foods that fall into the acid/alkaline categories in mind is helpful to making food choices:

- ◆ Strongly acid foods include meat, fish and soft, carbonated drinks like colas
- ◆ Mildly acid foods include grains, legumes, nuts
- ◆ Mildly alkaline foods include fruits, berries, vegetables, dairy
- ◆ Strongly alkaline foods include green leafy vegetable, spinach, broccoli

Soft, carbonated drinks that contain a massive amount of sugar are worth a special mention, because they also contain phosphorous, and have a pH of around 2.8 – which is highly acidic. Cut them out immediately as they are so detrimental to your health.

Good hydration is also essential for maintaining alkaline balance of the body. Where the mineral content of the water is good, and contains calcium and magnesium, it will be alkaline and drinking adequate quantities helps enormously by not only re-alkalinising the body, but also helping to neutralise toxins ready for elimination. Water that has more oxygen atoms and fewer hydrogen atoms, like distilled water or reverse osmosis water, is more alkaline. More hydrogen makes water acidic, but if water is neutralised it can help reduce acidic waste.

In addition, for the body to try and normalise any highly acidic state, calcium is leached from the bones, creating a potential weakness there and depleting the body further of critical nutrients, and removing the body's reserves for this purpose rather than in support of reproduction.

TAKING VITAMIN AND MINERAL SUPPLEMENTS

Taking vitamin and mineral supplements should not be necessary, unless advised by your doctor or if you feel your diet has been inadequate over a long period of time. And bear in mind that, although processed foods might be less nutritionally beneficial than fresh foods, they usually have added vitamins. Just look at the list of vitamins added to the humble cornflake! The important thing here is balance. Taking a daily dose of multivitamins is unlikely to do you much harm, but if you suddenly start taking excessive quantities of say, zinc (because you have read somewhere that it helps malnour-ished rats to conceive), you could affect the iron uptake of your body. So taking more than you need of one vitamin or mineral is not beneficial. You only need traces of these minerals and this is easily had from a diverse diet as outlined above. It is easy to be seduced by the marketing of some vitamin and mineral combinations, those designed for 'mums-to-be', so take them if it makes you feel better but do not imagine that they will be some sort of cure-all. Of course every mother-to-be wants to give their child the best possible start in life, which is what this marketing trades on, and many women consider it a relatively harmless sort of insurance policy.

The only supplement that is highly recommended prior to con-ception, and for the first few of months of pregnancy, is folic acid. Department of Health guidelines suggest a daily dose of 0.4 mg prior to conception and for at least the first three months. Folic acid is known to have a link in reducing the incidence of spina bifida and other neural tube defects in babies and will certainly be advised if you have had a previous baby with this congenital defect. Natural sources for folic acid include leafy green vegetables – spinach, broccoli and brussel sprouts – and also Marmite, potatoes and oranges. Folic acid is also one of the B group of vitamins, so is very often added to fortified breads and cereals.

While folic acid supplements are available on prescription, prescription charges are made until you are *actually* pregnant, after which they are free. And, given that prescription charges are more than the cost of purchasing it yourself, you may as well just buy it.

The other thing to bear in mind about spina bifida is that its cause is described as multi-factorial – that is, it can be caused by many things. So even if you take folic acid as recommended, you will still be checked during early pregnancy for your levels of blood alpha-fetoprotein, which could indicate that your baby has spina bifida. What is known is that women who have had one baby with spina bifida can reduce the incidence of any subsequent baby suffering it by 70% if they take folic acid supplements prior to, and during early pregnancy.

Recent research from the American *Nurses' Health Study* looked at the dietary intake of Omega3 essential fatty acids, found in oily fish, among 70,709 women. It found that those women who had the highest dietary intake of Omega3 EFAs were 22 percent less likely to be diagnosed with endometriosis, and all the health and fertility problems that can involve. Bear in mind, however, that if you choose to supplement with Omega3 you should choose a pharmaceutical grade product with high levels of Omega3 EPA and DHA, so just taking a dose of cod liver oil won't be sufficient.

In another study, the fat-soluble vitamin, vitamin D, was shown to be implicated in a study of infertile women carried out by Yale University Medical School in 2008. Of the sixty-seven infertile women who participated, only seven percent of them had normal vitamin D levels, while the rest had either insufficient levels or clinical deficiency and this was particularly marked in women with ovulatory disturbances and also those with polycystic ovary syndrome. Dietary intake comes from full-fat sources, plus eggs and oily fish, but the body also requires regular exposure to sunlight, but it can be difficult to obtain enough from the diet to make a therapeutic difference. However, when considering supplementation, again–take expert advice.

If for some reason you, or your doctor, feel you would benefit from an analysis of your nutritional needs, perhaps to identify any nutritional deficiencies that may be relevant both to general health and to specific problems with conception, this is possible through specialist laboratories like the Biolab Medical Unit (see Useful Addresses). Any referrals have to be made through either a medical doctor, registered osteopath or registered chiropractor. These nutritional profiles do not come cheap so you may find some resistance from your NHS doctor, and you may have to offer to pay yourself or seek help on this privately.

While most people have a more than nutritionally adequate diet, for some experiencing problems in conception and successful pregnancy, a closer look at what is eaten, in association with other considerations, may be well worthwhile. The correlation between good nutrition and successful pregnancy has been examined at length by the organisation Foresight, the Association for the Promotion of Pre-Conceptual Care (see Useful Addresses) and certainly a number of their research studies suggest that improved nutrition can make a difference. Foresight can be contacted direct for information and advice, and there is a network of local branches throughout the UK and some overseas.

WEIGHT

Another aspect of what we eat is what we weigh. Obesity has a definite impact on problems with ovulation, and if this is the case then treating women with fertility problems who are overweight is more difficult, and they run greater risks from the treatment itself. Obesity can also mean that women respond less well to medication, and that rates of miscarriage are increased. Ovulation disorders can often be simply rectified through weight loss, without the need for medical intervention. Some infertility clinics may not offer treatment where a woman is classified as obese, until weight loss is achieved. Very often this assessment is based on an individual's body mass index (BMI), where a woman's weight is divided by the square of her height (kilograms/metres squared). Acceptable BMIs range from 20 to 25, and anything over 30 is considered to be obese.

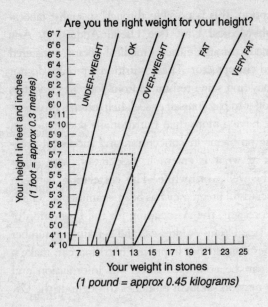

Height/weight chart (source: HEA)

Being underweight can also create problems with ovulation, and this is clearly seen in anorexic women who cease to ovulate and have periods. This can also occur through excessive exercise – a lot of female athletes cease ovulating when training very hard. However, both these instances are extremes – designed merely to emphasise the point that a sensible approach to weight, weight loss and exercise is required. If you are becoming obsessional about it, it will not do you much good!

Check out your height/weight profile from the chart below and, if you think your weight may be contributing to a problem with conception, discuss this with your doctor. If there are recommendations to be made about weight loss, or weight gain, that are relevant to you for conception, then your doctor cannot only give you the most specific advice, but he or she can also refer you to a dietician or even to a pre-conception clinic (if one exists in your area) for help, advice and support.

WEIGHT-LOSS DIETS

If you find yourself in the FAT or VERY FAT section of the chart, hormone production and fertility can also be affected because oestrogen is produced from fat cells, and the more fat cells, the more oestrogen. Excess weight can create an excess of oestrogen, which will put the delicate hormonal balance out especially with regard to progesterone. Progesterone rises when oestrogen levels drop after ovulation, and is responsible for helping conception, implantation and the continued thick lining of the womb necessary for the initial stability and growth of the fetal embryo. If oestrogen levels stay high, then there is no stimulus for the secretion of progesterone, which is so essential for pregnancy to occur and continue.

However, while losing excess weight is advantageous, going on an extreme weight-loss diet could be counter-productive, as many of these are based on excluding whole food groups, ie. carbohydrates. You should also be aware that a weight-loss diet that totally excludes a food group will inevitably exclude some nutrient sources that your body needs. In addition, a weight-loss diet like the Atkins diet has a tendency to make the body very acidic, because of the high intake of protein. An acidic environment is not ideal when it comes to conception (see pages 39–40).

If you're serious about improving your eating habits in such a way that will help you lose weight, you could do worse than follow what has become known as the GI diet. The Glycaemic Index is a measure of how fast the carbohydrate in your food is converted into your blood sugar. Foods that have a high GI rating are those that quickly raise the blood sugar level, and an insulin level to match, resulting in yo-yoing blood sugar levels, which can result in feeling hungry again within a couple of hours, and in need of a sugar 'fix' (check out www.glycemicindex.com for more information). Remember too that high GI foods also use up other nutrients during digestion, and a diet high in refined sugars could leave you short of the B group of vitamins, for example.

What you need is to eat foods that have a low GI, which take longer to get into the system, and which don't cause inappropriate surges of insulin. Complex carbohydrates are one such group of foods with a low GI, like porridge oats, buckwheat, wholewheat pastas or spaghetti, pulses like kidney beans, lentils and baked beans (choose low-sugar), and remember that potatoes have a higher GI index if baked than if chipped, because the fat in which chips are cooked reduces digestion time. If you include an exercise routine as part of your weight-loss plan, exercise coaches also recommend exercising around two hours after eating, allowing time for carbohydrate conversion to occur. This way, you will burn fat cells rather than muscle cells for energy – which is better for both energy and weight loss.

Breakfast is the most important meal of the day as it kick-starts your metabolism, and the higher your metabolic rate the more calories you'll burn. No breakfast and your metabolic rate remains sluggish. If you're serious about weight loss, boost your metabolic rate by eating a breakfast of complex carbohydrate, and include some protein to help stabilize your blood-sugar levels: a boiled egg and slice of wholemeal toast with freshly-squeezed orange juice is perfect, although porridge or buckwheat is a good alternative.

EXERCISE

Generally speaking, few of us do anything like enough regular exercise and most of us would see immediate benefit from increasing what little we do take. An optimum of regular exercise is really very little: twenty minutes three times a week. Exercise helps keep the body in good working order, and can help in reducing weight gain. It has long-term benefits in helping prevent coronary heart disease, high blood pressure, diabetes and osteoporosis. It is also psychologically beneficial because it helps concentration and relieves stress. Whatever form of exercise you choose to do regularly, it should increase your breathing and heart rate for a period. In a busy schedule introducing exercise can seem problematic so look at ways it can be incorporated naturally: walk rather than take the car for local journeys; get off the bus one stop earlier; use the stairs rather than the lift; while also looking at ways in which you can take more formal exercise regularly.

However, while most of us do not take enough exercise to be beneficial to health, there are some who over-exercise. Very vigorous, regular exercise can actually inhibit ovulation in women, and may also affect sperm production in men. This is most relevant for athletes, or others in specific training, but visiting the gym every day for an hour's demanding work-out, or running long distances every other day, may be enough to affect a susceptible individual. If a woman has irregular periods and a vigorous exercise regime, cutting down may help over a period of time. Balancing exercise may be better: some working-out combined with regular yoga sessions, for example.

SMOKING

There is no way round this one: smoking will damage your health. Smoking is also more detrimental for women's general health than for men's. It increases the risk of cervical cancer, the tendency to reach menopause earlier and the likelihood of osteoporosis. While there is no proven link between smoking and failure to conceive, it is heavily implicated in miscarriage.

Recent research from Radboud University in the Netherlands, published in March 2005, followed 8,000 women whose average age was thirty-two who were in the process of trying to conceive using IVF. The birth rate among women who smoked was 28% lower than among non-smokers, and the rate of miscarriage among smokers was higher. The conclusion was that, in terms of outcome, smoking added ten years to the chronological age of a woman trying to conceive. This may not seem much of a problem for a woman in her early twenties who is trying to conceive, but if you are in your thirties, there can be no better indication that stopping smoking will improve your chances.

For men who produce sperm of variable quality, smoking can have quite an impact on sperm production. The more heavily you smoke, the worse the effect, although even light, regular smoking is not good for you. Give up and get help to do so if necessary: your local health centre may run a smoking cessation clinic, or contact QUIT, the free national helpline for smokers (see Useful Addresses).

Even if you do not have much of a commitment to your own health, bear in mind that the children of adults who smoke have a far greater chance of becoming smokers themselves. In addition, children brought up in homes where smoking occurs have a greater risk of glue-ear disease and chest infections. Babies of mothers who smoke tend to be of a lower birthweight, too. So for your child's sake, if not your own, there are very strong reasons why you should stop.

'I couldn't imagine not smoking, and continued to have the occasional cigarette during my pregnancy although, officially, I had stopped. I had no intention of stopping altogether and assumed I would start again after the birth. But when our daughter was born, she was so beautiful and perfect that the idea of us, or anyone else, smoking around her seemed wrong. So we both gave up – and easily. Besides, there wasn't much time for a cigarette in the early weeks!'

Jutta, aged 36

'I consciously decided to give up before trying to get pregnant – and it was hard! But, after I had got over the craving, I felt so much better for it. And my appetite returned – I really enjoy my food now, which is an unexpected bonus. And I sleep much better too. Being pregnant doesn't feel so daunting now I feel so much healthier, either.'

Clare, aged 27

ALCOHOL

An occasional alcoholic drink will not do you much harm, and could even be beneficial. Regular, moderate drinking is probably safe too and the recommended guidelines for weekly intake are fourteen units for women, and twenty-one units for men. A unit equals half a pint of ordinary strength beer, lager or cider; a single measure of wine; or a single measure of spirits. However, even this 'recommended' amount, if drunk regularly, may have an adverse effect on your general health over a period of time and could increase your risk of stroke, some cancers and coronary artery disease. Women are more affected by alcohol than men, and this effect can vary during different times of the month, and some women are more affected than others.

Heavy drinking is definitely bad for your health and can have quite serious implications for fertility, particularly in men. Excessive alcohol intake can depress sperm production, thus reducing sperm count. Again, as with smoking, if the number of sperm being produced are high this might not matter much, but with low, or variable, sperm quantities it may be crucial. In addition, there is no doubt that excess drinking affects a man's sexual performance, and causes impotency in some men, which has an obvious and direct result on a couple's ability to conceive! And for women who have a history of miscarriage, then a look at alcohol intake may be particularly relevant, as studies have shown there to be a definite connection.

Excessive drinking also influences what you eat, and you may find that your diet is suffering because you do not feel hungry, or cannot be bothered to cook. Your sleep may be affected too. Many people who drink have disturbed sleep patterns that can leave you feeling unwell. So drinking can have a direct impact on your general health in the short-term, as well as in the long-term, which, for those trying to conceive, could be unhelpful.

While it is difficult to be prescriptive about exactly how much one should or should not drink, if you are having any problems with conceiving it might be wise to take a look at how much you are drinking during the course of a week, and possibly cut down. Or maybe cut out spirits, and just have a glass of wine with your evening meal. Unless there are very specific recommendations, perhaps on the advice of your doctor, there does not seem to be much point in giving up completely but there is also no reason to drink to the limit of the recommendations outlined above. Of course, giving up alcohol completely for a period of time might make you feel better about your efforts to help yourself, in which case do so, but not if it leaves you feeling resentful about what you are having to do in order to successfully conceive.

Once you are pregnant, you may decide to err on the side of absolute caution and give up alcohol for the duration of your pregnancy. Or you may decide not to drink during the first three months. Some women decide to give up spirits but continue to enjoy the occasional glass of beer or wine. As long as you avoid excessive amounts of alcohol, and binge-drinking, the occasional drink is unlikely to do your unborn baby much harm. But this is entirely up to you, and if you feel unsure about it, talk to your midwife or doctor. They will be able to advise you about what is right for you, and put your mind at rest about any issues to do with drinking alcohol in pregnancy that may concern you.

AGE

Most of what is relevant about age in couples wanting to conceive is primarily relevant to women. There is some decline in a man's ability to produce sperm as his age advances, although this is also influenced by his general health. There is, however, copious reference made in our society to the female 'biological clock'. Focus has been concentrated on this in recent years because of the general trend for women to delay having children until their late twenties and early thirties.

This may be for a number of reasons, the most commonly cited is that working women want to have achieved something in work, or be established in their careers before taking time out to have babies. It may also be that current expectations of what is needed to financially support a family, and the economic climate in which we are attempting to do this, make couples less secure about starting their family. A woman's expectation about her relationship with her partner may not be as solid as in the past, and in an attempt to find a relationship secure enough to avoid being left 'holding the baby', delays occur. Who knows exactly why, but most women are aware that there is some pressure on them to have a baby, should they want one, before it is 'too late'.

NEW STATISTICS

Figures from the UK's Office for National Statistics, published in 2009, showed that over half of all babies (54%) born in 2008 were born to mothers aged 25–34, while 25% were born to mothers aged below 25 years, and 20% to mothers aged 35 plus. The average age at which a mother gave birth remained the same from 29.3 years in 2002 and 29.4 years in 2003, and 29.3 years in 2008, while the average age of a woman having her first baby was 27.4 years. While the majority of women have their babies during their late twenties and early thirties, there shows a continuing trend towards older women continuing to have babies.

1993			
All births	**35 +**	**40 +**	**45 +**
673,467	58,824	9,985	539
2003			
621,469	97,386	18,205	875
2008			
708,711	116,220	24,991	1,428

(Source: Office for National Statistics)

What is known is that there is also a general decline in fertility as a woman gets older and progresses towards that natural cessation of female fertility, menopause. This can be for a number of reasons:

- ovulation in the older woman can become irregular, so reducing the number of opportunities for conception;
- there is an increased possibility for genetic defect, and miscarriage, because of the age of the ovaries;
- an older women is more likely to have fibroids, or other problems with the lining of the womb, which can make implantation of a fertilised egg difficult;
- frequency of love-making may decline, reducing the possibilities for conception.

All of this can make depressing reading, especially as anyone over the age of thirty-five is considered 'older' when it comes to fertility. One benefit of being so 'old' is that you are recommended to seek help with problems with conceiving after only six months. Although you may never need medical help, it is an opportunity to check things over with a doctor and, in most cases, be reassured, or get the ball rolling if needs be. But be warned, doctors can hold very different views on what timing is relevant and this may be influenced by availability of resources in your area. Each health trust makes its own decisions about the infertility services it chooses to provide, and its policies about referral and treatment will differ. It can sometimes appear to be some sort of lottery based on your post code, which is often not far from the truth. In actuality it is to do with the allocation of funding for these services, by your local health trust, that influences what is available.

Ovarian reserve test

This test is designed to assess both the number of immature eggs in the ovaries, and also their quality – which gives an indication of a woman's potential fertility. It works by detecting the levels of three female hormones, using a blood sample taken on day three of her menstrual cycle (that is, the third day of her period). The three hormones tested for are FSH (follicle stimulating hormone), AMH (anti-Müllerein hormone), and Inhibin B. As a woman's ovaries start to fail, she produces high levels of FSH, in an attempt to stimulate the ovarian follicles to produce an egg. Inhibin B is also produced by the ovaries, in response to the stimulation and maturation of an egg follicle, which serves to inhibit the production of FSH, so that only one follicle is stimulated at a time. If the ovaries are not working well, you can expect a high level of FSH and a low level of Inhibin B and AMH.

'I couldn't believe it when my doctor told me not to worry and just keep on trying. We had been 'trying' for three years, with no result at all, and I was thirty-three then. I felt very anxious that we should get the ball rolling, and eventually had a check-up privately.'

Amrit, aged 37

'My doctor was brilliant. He took the time to listen to our concerns which, in retrospect, were mainly panic, given I was only twenty-nine. He made an appointment with the specialist, but in the meantime put me in touch with an NFP teacher who was very helpful in teaching me about my own fertility cycle. Needless to say we never needed the appointment with the specialist – I was pregnant before it came through!

Sara, aged 32

However, if you are having regular periods, making love frequently and are in good health, you need not presume that you will have problems *just* because you have crossed some magic chronological line. Because successful conception is dependent on a variety of factors, age alone is only one of a number of contributing factors that may need to be considered if you are trying to conceive.

And it is worth thinking about the following: in 1950 26,017, 40-somethings gave birth, while in 1994 there were only 10,729 births in the same age group. And given that we are somehow 'younger' at 40 than our parents were, and potentially healthier and fitter, late pregnancy – as long as conception occurs – should not be a problem. All sorts of high-profile women – Susan Sarandon, Kim Basinger, Goldie Hawn, Jane Seymour, Patricia Hodge, David Bowie's wife, Iman and Cherie Blair to name a few – have successfully given birth in their forties. Any pregnancy in a woman over the age of thirty-five is considered, medically, somehow more 'risky', but with good antenatal care the risks can be minimised and a healthy pregnancy can be enjoyed.

One last word on age. Bear in mind that IVF outcomes are significantly less good, the older the mother. HFEA national data in 2010 showed that only 24% of all IVF cycles result in a birth. This drops to 12% for women aged 40–42, and only 3% of women aged 43–44 have a successful outcome from IVF.

ENVIRONMENTAL HAZARDS

Environmental hazards are regularly cited in the press as becoming more prevalent, and having an effect on health. Fortunately, our bodies are well-equipped to deal with a certain level of toxic load, but it's when this is exceeded, or when other elements of our health are compromised, then exposure to these levels might be worth considering, and where they might be coming from.

Working with chemicals, for example in printing or hairdressing, may be an obvious example. And attention has been focused on those chemicals that are routinely used in toiletries, personal hygiene and beauty care products, from preservatives in moisturisers to formaldehyde in nail polish hardeners, because of their possible toxicity. This may not cause any sort of a reaction, but formaldehyde is highly toxic, a carcinogen, neurotoxic and genotoxic (can affect genetic material) and over time could place an additional demand on the liver, the body's organ of detoxification, depleting your natural resources and ability to keep the body clear of the rest of the toxins you might be exposed to – it's all a question of toxic load, and how your body deals with it.

Although most chemicals in regular use are passed OK, it's the incessant exposure to the use of one or more products over long periods of time that can create problems. It has been estimated that the average women who wears lipstick regularly, will eat two pounds of lipstick in her lifetime, the content of which is based on petrol by-products! Large manufacturers need to create products with a shelf life of up to ten years, to make the profit margins high enough for their company shareholders, and use strong chemical preservatives to do so, but at a possible risk of your health. Using a moisturiser once a month would create no problem, but using the same product – complete with chemical preservatives – twice a day, for years, could possibly be a different story.

Some chemical preservatives, known as parabens, are found in most moisturisers for both women and men and are known to chemically imitate oestrogens, which can cause hormonal imbalances. These in turn may make the difference to ovulation, implantation or even sperm quality and quantity, in susceptible people. Foundation make-ups, which many women wear every day, also have a high level of parabens, according to the Women's Environmental Network (from whom more information is available). Many toothpastes contain the anti-bacterial agent triclosan, a very persistent chemical that has been found in breast milk, which gives some indication of its ability to get into the body. There have been cases of its contamination with dioxin, an extremely toxic substance, too, and some evidence to suggest that triclosan can degrade into dioxin when it gets into the environment.

Shaving creams, used by many men every day, can contain a substance called diethylhexyl adipate (DEHA) along with its parabens, which has been linked to cancerous tumours in mice and abnormal embryos in rats. Propylene gylcol, a major component of soap products, can depress the central nervous system. Sun protection creams, which we are advised to slap on in large quantities, several times a day, are also under question because of the quantities of hormone-mimicking chemicals they contain. One environmental toxologist, Dr Margret Schlumpf at the University of Zurich, has gone so far as to suggest that pregnant and lactating women should avoid their use.

In the same way that we became more conscious of chemical additives and preservatives finding their way into our foods, so many people are taking to checking the labels on their personal hygiene and beauty products, from tampons to hair dye. As a rule of thumb, the more chemical ingredients listed on the product's contents, the better it is to avoid it, and even those products that are requently used and should be OK, like lanolin, may be contaminated by chemicals like DDT.

Check for the following on the labels of products you buy:

Parabens
    Benzophenone-3
    Butyl Benzyl Phthalate
    Butylated Hydroxyanisole (BHA)
    Butlymethoxydibenzoylmethane (B-MDM)
    Dibtyl Phthalate
    Diethyl Phthalate
    Homosalate (HMS)
    Methyl-benzylidene Camphor (4-MBC)
    Octyl-dimethyl-PABA (OD-PABA)
    Octyl-methoxycinnamate (OMC)
    Resorcinol

Formaldehyde precursors
    Diazolidinyl Urea
    DMDM-Hydantoin
    Imidazolidinyl Urea

Metheneamine
Quaternium-15
Sodium Hydroxymethylglycinate

For further checklists, go to the Greenpeace or Women's Environmental Network sites (www.greenpeace.org.uk, www.wen.org.uk).

VAGINAL LUBRICANTS

Over the last thirty years, several studies have found that all vaginal lubricants studied to date contain sperm damaging properties that reduce sperm motility (the ability of sperm to move) as well as sperm viability (the amount of live sperm per ejaculate).

One study reviewed sixteen lubricants and their effects on sperm health, including all the leading brands of vaginal lubricants and found that they all had a negative effect on sperm motility as well as viability, even when used in tiny quantities of less than ten percent. In fact, it was found that the spermicidal quality of some products was comparable to contraceptive gels. Another negative effect was that the ability of sperm to move through the cervix, into the womb, was also reduced.

Even water-soluble vaginal lubricants are damaging to sperm health because they contain glycerin and propylene glycol, both of which are extremely hyperosmotic (absorb water). This is damaging to sperm, which is highly sensitive to adverse osmolality (concentration of particles that are osmotically active in a solution). In fact, both high and low levels of osmolality can cause sperm cells to shrink or swell excessively. Sperm motility also decreases with high osmolality. On average, vaginal lubricants have osmolality levels that are between three to ten times that of semen, thereby resulting in irreversible damage to sperm motility when used. In addition, the pH levels in vaginal lubricants are quite low, which also damages sperm. According to the World Health Organization (WHO), healthy pH levels for sperm range from 7.0 to 8.5, a level that is consistent with female cervical mucus at the time of ovulation. So, if a vaginal lubricant has a pH level that is lower than 7, it will create an acid environment that is damaging to sperm.

The good news is that there is a range of organic, alkaline, baby friendly products new to the market, one of which is optimistically called Yes, Yes, Yes (see Useful Addresses).

STRESS

Although there is some argument to suggest that stress can be a factor in infertility, and we may know of or have experienced times when working hard, studying, or even moving house has played havoc with our menstrual cycle, stress and anxiety are more likely to be the consequence of infertility, and infertility treatments, rather than the cause of it. Women conceive quite successfully under amazingly stressful circumstances, starvation, war or worse, so being stressed is not, in itself, a reason why conception does not occur. And the National Association of Natural Family Planning Teachers has found that stress was a causative factor in pregnancy among women using NFP methods to try and avoid conception!

Measuring individual levels of stress is both subjective and imprecise, and its possible effect difficult to quantify. Certainly if you feel anxious and stressed, it is worth taking steps to try and alleviate it if only because life is just so much easier without feeling strung out as well. Numerous symptoms of stress compound the situation, making you feel physically worse: insomnia, lack of appetite, palpitations, for example, although not serious in themselves, can undermine how you feel you are coping. Making sure you eat well, get adequate rest and relaxation, attend to any minor health complaints and try not to feel at odds with your body which, you may feel, has somehow let you down.

One of the problems with stress is that it is self-perpetuating, not least because of the physical symptoms that can arise. Reassuring yourself these physical symptoms will subside once the cause of your stress is resolved can become increasingly difficult and, if so, you may want to take steps to counteract these feelings. This may mean taking a holiday, having a regular massage, seeking a counsellor or just taking up some regular activity that takes your mind off things for a while. While these suggestions may seem simplistic, having a personal stress-buster campaign may prevent events spiralling while giving you the resources to cope. And if you do have problems with conception, then keeping a sense of perspective, while finding out all you can, is beneficial.

'I couldn't believe the palpitations I had when I managed to convince myself I'd never conceive a baby. I was quite certain I had some heart problem. Once I realised what was going on, I started going to a yoga class recommended by a friend. Just concentrating on gently exercising, and relaxing, really helped. I continued with these classes throughout my pregnancy, too.'

Sally, aged 40

'Work was unbelievably difficult. My mum was pressurising me about having children. Jeff was endlessly telling me to slow down and ease up. I felt pressurised from all sides and inside my head was a little voice saying, you'll never get pregnant in this state. I really began to suspect the worst when the littlest thing reduced me to tears. It then turned out that I was actually three weeks' pregnant – I thought my period was late because of the stress I was under, not because I was pregnant!'

Angela, aged 37

Clinicians are by and large unequivocal: stress is not a causative factor in failure to conceive. Individual women and couples may tell a different story, but it can be reassuring to think that although you feel stressed, the actual impact on your ability to conceive is probably negligible. What may be more relevant is if a cause of the stress is some unreconciled feeling about getting pregnant in the first place. If you are deeply ambivalent about having a baby at all, or resistant to the idea of giving up your independence, or fearful about the responsibility a baby brings, or anxious about your partner's commitment, or even scared of the possible pain of giving birth, then these issues need addressing. They may be subconsciously holding you back. What makes it more difficult is that you may not even be aware that there are reasons like these behind the feelings of stress you are experiencing. Whatever the clinicians may say, the mind-body link is very strong, although it may not be the stress itself – but the reasons behind it – that need examining.

If you have any reason to think this is the case, then you need to talk it through with someone objective. A trained counsellor can be extremely useful – even just for a few sessions – while you try and sort this out, if needs be. Your GP or health centre may be able to advise you, or contact Relate, either through your local telephone directory or their head office (see Useful Addresses). Private counsellors also exist and are probably best consulted after personal recommendation. This need not be a long-term commitment to psychoanalysis, but the benefit of structuring your thoughts with the help of an expert can be invaluable.

'The idea of having a baby was fine, but the idea of parenting a child with Mike was – it turned out – making me feel very ambivalent about getting pregnant at all. It took me ages to work out that this was why I was feeling so worried about everything. Eventually we saw a Relate counsellor who helped me sort out my feelings. Mike had had no idea about how I'd been feeling, he had just been trying to be very cool and low-key to take the pressure off me. The more stressed I became, the more distant he appeared to be. I just assumed he had changed his mind about having children with me, but I was too scared to ask him about it. Thank goodness we sorted it out! Sophy was born eighteen months later, and we've since had two more.'

Karen, aged 36

5 Difficulties in conception

'Having spent so much of my life trying not to get pregnant, it hadn't occurred to me that conceiving a baby would be a problem. Initially I didn't worry, but after a year and a bit of thinking it would happen I began to panic that there was something badly wrong. Thankfully, Simon was very calm about it all and, when it turned out that I wasn't always ovulating – which explained my slightly haphazard cycles – we knew we would have to think a little more carefully about how we were going about it. What I did find useful were those ovulation predictor tests, at least I knew when I was about to ovulate – if I was going to – and that helped. Finally our first baby was born, and we are now trying for another.'

Anne, aged 33

'I always thought I might have a problem conceiving because I'd had an ectopic pregnancy some years ago, and one of my tubes was blocked as a consequence. But, in the end, it didn't seem to make much difference. I was pregnant within six months of trying.'

Lucy, aged 29

Lots of couples have difficulties in conceiving, but most are successful in the end. It is worth remembering that around half of sexually active couples take up to six months or more to conceive, and the average chance of conceiving in any one month is only around one in four or five. One in six couples have some difficulty in conceiving, and about one in ten need some help. About one third of couples attending fertility clinics go on to successfully have a baby, while many others get what help they need just by visiting their family doctor. Although accurate, these figures only represent those who seek help. There may be many others with fertility problems about which nothing is known, because there will always be some couples who say nothing and others who never seek help.

The term secondary infertility refers to current infertility where there has been a previous pregnancy, whether or not the pregnancy has gone to term and a baby was born. Around half of all infertile couples seeking treatment have problems with secondary infertility. Few couples are actually infertile, although many may be referred to as subfertile, taking more than one year to conceive. None of these descriptions will necessarily mean much when you are tackling the problem yourself, but it is useful to know what doctors mean by the terminology they use.

WHEN TO SEEK HELP

The general rules of thumb for when to suspect there is a problem for which you may need help are outlined below. In fact, unless you fulfil one or other of these criteria, you may be told to carry on trying and wait a while longer. This is because it is within the normal range for couples to take up to a year to conceive, so unless there is a specific problem, anticipate only passing support or advice initially. Remember also that policies on what is and what is not available vary quite dramatically, depending on the health authority or trust where you live. Some will not fund any treatment at all for women over the age of thirty-five, for example, and because treatment times can be lengthy, in some cases, taking several years, it is as well to be aware of this.

However, see your doctor if you are trying to conceive a baby and any of the following apply:

- if you are both under the age of thirty, and have been having unprotected intercourse for eighteen months without getting pregnant;
- if you are a woman aged between thirty and thirty-five and have been having unprotected intercourse for a year with no luck (although the Infertility Network recommend contacting your doctor after only six months, because of the possibility of a cut-off age of thirty-five in your area);
- if you are a woman aged over thirty-five, see your doctor if after six months of unprotected intercourse there is no pregnancy;
- if you have problems with your periods, they are irregular, painful, heavy or absent;
- if you have had any gynaecological infections in the past, or have had a burst appendix;
- if you find sexual intercourse painful in any way.

And in men, it is worth checking out the following:

- history of mumps, or other infection which resulted in inflamed testicles;
- any history of sexually transmitted disease like gonorrhoea;
- undescended testicle(s);
- problems with intercourse, for example with sustaining an erection or premature ejaculation;
- any repeated exposure to toxic chemicals or radiation.

The causes of infertility tend to occur in men in around one third of cases, in women in around one third of cases, and in the rest both the man and the woman are involved or there may be no apparent cause found. Some of the reasons for reduced fertility may be quite simple, and easily solved, for example the timing of intercourse. Apparently less than half the women in the UK know when they are most likely to get pregnant in any one cycle (and one can only hazard a guess at how many men know). As the opportunity to get pregnant occurs for only approximately three to five days during the woman's cycle, and the average couple only make love twice a week, you can immediately begin to see how important the timing of intercourse is if, for example, your twice a week occurred either side of the five days in which it might be possible to conceive.

One of the reasons suggested for difficulty in conceiving as women get older is that couples are, generally, making love less often. The truth of the matter is that the greater the number of times you make love, the greater the chances of conceiving. If, however, you are making love every day for months on end and not getting pregnant, then it is certainly feasible to think there may be a problem.

When considering why pregnancy is not happening, it is worth understanding what is necessary for conception to occur. This is covered in chapter two, The Female fertility cycle; but to recap briefly, conception requires the production of an egg, the availability of the male sperm, that they should meet successfully so that the egg is fertilised, and that this fertilised egg should successfully implant in the womb. If there is any failure at any of these stages, problems arise.

In women, problems may arise because of one or more of the following:

- ◆ ovulation does not occur, or only occurs haphazardly;
- ◆ a blockage in the fallopian tube through which the egg has to journey to meet the sperm;
- ◆ a problem in the womb, perhaps caused by endometriosis or fibroids, that prevents successful implantation;
- ◆ hormone deficiencies which may affect ovulation, production of cervical mucus and implantation;
- ◆ medication: one of the first questions any doctor will ask you is if you are taking any medication regularly, in case this has an effect on your fertility.

In the man, problems can arise through one or more of the following:

- quality and quantity of sperm produced;
- blockage in the tubes of the testes;
- problems with sustaining an erection and ejaculation.

And then there are problems which occur because of the specific combination of two individual partners. For example, if the man has a borderline sperm count and the woman ovulates haphazardly. Or perhaps if the woman produces antibodies to her partner's sperm, so that it is not able to survive the journey and fertilise the egg. Or if there is some sub-clinical infection present, one that produces no apparent symptoms, that has escaped diagnosis. Where there are a combination of factors causing a problem, the individual factor responsible may only be relatively minor so the possibilities for conception continue to exist. Very few people are completely infertile, although it may take time to locate the problem and find a solution.

'I just wish we hadn't waited so long before seeing our doctor. I think we were both trying to be very relaxed about it and low-key, assuming everything was fine. I kept on thinking how meaningless the tests we were having must be, because I refused to believe anything was wrong. It turned out that one of my tubes was completely blocked, and the other partially. I was devastated when I realised that our only option was IVF, and I really resented all the treatment necessary to get pregnant. In some ways, if I couldn't have a baby naturally I didn't want one at all. But I went through with it because I knew how much my partner wanted a baby. Of course, I'm glad now, but it was a difficult time.'

Tina, aged 34

'I was so sure something was wrong when, after four months, I still wasn't pregnant. I had got pregnant so quickly the first time, the minute we decided we wanted to have a baby I got pregnant. So I couldn't believe it when the doctor told me it was much too early to worry. But, as Jason pointed out,

we just weren't having as much sex now as we had been having the first time! Of course it wasn't going to happen immediately. I mean, we weren't doing it every night any more, it was more like twice a week!'

Janet, aged 29

IMMUNE PROBLEMS

Immunity is a highly complex subject, and it's not really known why an inappropriate response by a woman's immune system should occur when trying to conceive, or why it appears to be occurring with greater frequency. However, an inappropriate immune response seems likely to be more common in women who have some degree of long-term immune system activity, perhaps because of a history of endometriosis, or PCOS, or even migraines – all of which have placed a long standing demand on the immune system. In addition, the delayed onset of conception – women waiting until they are much older than before – may further complicate matters. Like any other body system, the immune system will be affected to some degree by its age. It even seems possible that if a couple have a tissue type that is very similar, this can confuse the woman's immune system into thinking that the developing embryo is a bunch of mutating 'self' cells, like cancer, which need to be destroyed.

All of this is further complicated by a degree of division within the medical establishment about what is and what isn't a result of an immune response, and how to treat its impact on fertility. What is known, however, is that some women's bodies respond to their partner's sperm as if it were an antigen, and even to a developing embryo. Having happened once, the situation is further complicated by the woman's immune system 'remembering' the antigen – her partner's sperm, or the developing embryo – making subsequent attempts at conception unsuccessful.

Understanding the way the immune system works, and how it can work inappropriately, is useful before trying to work out what the solutions might be. What is crucial is that the immune system should be balanced, and this is the key to restoring normal activity rather than trying to suppress its abnormal activity. Where a problem exists, it's largely a problem of hyper-activity of the system, which is trying too hard to deal with dangers that don't exist. Re-balancing, through lifestyle changes, improved nutrition, and reduction of environmental pollutants, will all help.

Dr Alan Beer, who has studied immune problems in pregnancy for over thirty years, and runs the Center for Reproductive Immunology and Genetics in Chicago (www.repro-med.net), has identified five main categories of immune problems that can cause inability to conceive, pregnancy loss and IVF failure. The level of severity runs from Category 1 to Category 5, with the latter being the most severe.

Category 1

This occurs when both parents' body cells are too similar, and the woman's body doesn't produce the blocking antibody necessary for her body to accept the developing embryo for implantation, so no placental cells begin to develop. As a consequence, the embryo dies. The existence of a Category 1 problem can lead to the stimulation of Categories 2 to 5.

Category 2

Repeated miscarriages, IVF failure, endometriosis or anything else that can lead to chronic tissue damage, resulting in a sustained immune response, can result in the production of antibodies to phospholipids. Under normal circumstances phospholipids exist in cell membranes, but under the stress caused by tissue damage, the production of what are called antiphospholipid antibodies occurs. These antibodies damage cell function making them behave inappropriately, resulting in inflammation and blood clotting abnormalities, which inevitably causes chaos in early pregnancy.

Category 3

In this category, women make antibodies to DNA or DNA by-products. DNA is the building block of genetic activity, and during the early cell division of an embryo's life genetic material from the sperm and the egg is being exchanged and incorporated into the embryo. The presence of these anti-DNA antibodies, identifiable through extensive blood testing at specialist clinics, cause inflammation around the embryo, or within the placenta, at the point at which implantation should occur, preventing the pregnancy from continuing.

Category 4

Here, a woman produces antibodies to her partner's sperm. The production of anti-sperm antibodies is associated with production of antiphospholipid antibodies (Category 2). Once a woman has produced these antibodies, they are effective against all sperm and aren't partner specific.

Category 5

This is the most complicated category of immune problems, involving natural killer cells. In spite of their name, natural killer cells are one of the thirty different types of lymphocytes of the immune system, and are present in the uterine lining. Under normal circumstances, there is a lot of antibody activity in the uterus, as the lining is shed each month during a period, keeping everything functioning well. Normal activity by natural killer cells during early pregnancy includes the release of cytokines that promote implantation and the formation of the placenta. Kept in balance by other body systems, like circulating hormones, natural killer cells are beneficial and designed to work for us rather than against us. However, if these go haywire, excessive release of cytokines causes damage to a developing embryo and placental cells, and the pregnancy fails.

When you consider these five categories, which are more complex than explained here, it becomes easier to understand how immune problems in pregnancy can build. An initial immune response, for example Category 1, may be enough to trigger a further immune response giving rise to another category. It's not unusual for a woman to have problems in more than one category.

Treatment for immune problems, once the category of problem has been successfully identified, can be very effective. This can be done by the use of low-dose steroids to suppress immune activity, taking a mild anti-coagulant daily to reduce blood clotting, or anti-TNF (tumour necrosis factor) therapy – but each treatment protocol must follow proper identification of the immune response that is giving rise to the problem.

Once it has been agreed between you and your doctor that, because conception has not occurred over a prescribed period of time, some investigations are necessary, you will be referred to a specialist doctor for this. This specialist doctor is most likely to be one with training in gynaecology, which is the branch of medicine concerned with female reproduction. He or she may also have additional training, expertise or interest in the area of infertility. However, unless you are referred to someone who runs an infertility clinic, you may find that there are limitations on the help available in your area, and you may subsequently be referred on. The commitment to specific infertility services within the NHS is known to be limited, so it really comes down to luck if the area in which you live is well served.

In addition, the types of investigative tests offered, and the order in which they may be carried out, will be influenced by a number of factors. First and foremost will be individual need, dependent on what is already known about a couple's fertility; second will be availability of specialist resources; and, finally, some decisions about what tests are pertinent will be linked to the specialist doctor's experience, expertise and working knowledge of the field. This last factor is perhaps the one in which there may be most variability. Suffice to say that the individual nature of your circumstances will influence, in part, what happens, and this should be borne in mind.

'I had no idea what a complicated procedure it was to try and get treated for infertility. Getting referred was only the first step. The clinic we were referred to was dependent on my local health authority agreeing to cover the cost of treatment, which they were not prepared to do at first. We had to really push for the help we needed.'

Hannah, aged 30

'When they told me what the NHS waiting list was like, I nearly died. I was already thirty-three, by the time we got to first base I would be past the cut-off date for treatment. We had no choice but to seek help privately and then it was only because my parents offered to help out financially.'

Gina, aged 37

'We had no problem, really. I mean, we had to wait six months for the initial appointment but after that we were accepted on a programme that reckoned to offer you three treatment cycles before reassessing you. I conceived the twins at our second attempt, which was lucky because I don't want to go through it again.'

Susie, aged 27

Your best source of information about what is available in the UK is from the Human Fertilisation and Embryology Authority (www.hfea.gov.uk), which produces a free, downloadable guide from their website. The HFEA is a regulatory body that makes sure all the 83 clinics in the UK comply with the law and provide safe and appropriate treatment. The HFEA also provides extremely comprehensive and up-to-date information on a range of issues, including:

- what treatment a clinic is licensed to carry out, ie. donor insemination, IVF, egg donation, ICSI, etc.
- success rates, ie. clinical pregnancy rates

- data on multiple births
- finding a clinic, and questions to ask

What help is provided for infertile couples by the NHS varies widely across the country. The NHS aims to provide at least one free cycle of IVF for women between the ages of 23 and 39, but this is also influenced by whether or not they meet the eligibility criteria. While the National Institute for Clinical Excellence (NICE) sets out fertility guidelines – and you can check these at www.nice.org.uk – other guidelines are determined locally, by the NHS organisation to which your GP refers you. It can be a bit of a lottery, and waiting lists can be long, and often the only alternative for couples is to go privately. The costs for this vary considerably, depending on what tests and treatments are recommended, and from clinic to clinic. However, typical costs for a cycle of IVF, including drugs and consultations can range between £4,000 to £8,000, and if you need specialised extras like egg donation or ICSI (intra-cycloplasmic sperm injection), it can cost more; while the cost of a single attempt at donor insemination can range from £500 to £1,000.

However, before you need to think about specialist treatment your doctor is probably able to carry out some preliminary checks and this may start with a routine look at your general health and sexual activity, perhaps with some recommendations on diet or exercise, and the timing of intercourse. He or she may also recommend some self-assessment of fertility awareness, perhaps temperature charting or cervical mucus symptoms. In addition to this, your doctor may also take a blood sample to check the post-ovulation levels of the hormone progesterone. If ovulation has occurred, about a week later the corpus luteum should be producing a high level of progesterone. This can be reassuring if it is able to confirm ovulation, perhaps in conjunction with indicators thrown up by charting temperature and mucus symptoms. However, the timing of this blood test is important because, taken too early or too late in the cycle, the progesterone levels will automatically appear low.

At the same time, if the man is referred for semen analysis, a couple will already have gone some way to establishing whether or not there is a problem with both ovulation and production of sperm. Because of the length of time (up to a year in some areas on the NHS, although immediate it private) it can take for referral appointments with a doctor specialising in infertility to come through, then it is useful to begin some preliminary checks with your GP. So do not be put off when there seems to be a delay in seeing a specialist: it is entirely appropriate for your GP to make these initial checks and referral for semen analysis, and it will save time in the long run.

Initial tests should always be carried out on both the man and the woman because, even if the semen analysis indicates a below-average sperm count, it would be wrong to rule out problems in the woman without checking. While a low sperm count may contribute to a problem, it might not be the whole story in a couple's inability to conceive. Many men with low sperm production father children quite successfully. It is worth pointing out that a man's sperm count may vary over time. One low sperm count may represent an illness suffered several months previously, and the man's usual sperm production could actually lie within the normal range.

'When we started on the road towards investigating our possible infertility, I felt very relaxed about it and what it might mean. But somehow, as we got past each test, and had numerous discussions with endless doctors, we had to take care not to let it take over our lives. We also agreed only to tell a select few friends – and not our families – about it until we knew what was what. This was purely because we didn't want everyone to be always asking about our 'problem'. Because we were both so clear about how we wanted to handle it together it was all right. But it still wasn't an easy time and I'm just really glad its over, and we managed to have a baby at all. I still shudder when I think about it all.'

Dee, aged 38

'Having accepted that we had a problem, and we needed help to have a baby, I didn't mind all the tests really. I mean, you wouldn't choose to spend your morning with your legs in stirrups, but there are worse things. I think it was telling my dad that things might take some time that was the most difficult. I think he was afraid he would never be a grandfather.'

Alex, aged 33

What shouldn't be underestimated is the impact on a couple's relationship of a possible diagnosis of infertility and referral for investigations. For many couples, having children together is one of the reasons they are together. There may have been an unspoken assumption that this would inevitably be a feature of their future life. If for some reason this looks like it might not be possible, then it throws all sorts of other aspects of their relationship into relief. Women may fear being left because they are 'unable' to give the man they love a child and, equally, a man may feel that he is an inadequate partner if he can't make the woman he loves pregnant and give her a child. Infertility, real or anticipated, raises questions concerning our assumptions about what constitutes a 'real' man or a 'real' woman. Ask any woman who has actively chosen not to have children and she will probably list a number of criticisms levelled at her about selfishness, unnaturalness and worse. Even if we only pay lip service to the true value of children in the society in which we live, it is a society that says we should want to have children. Indeed, it is written into the Christian marriage contract that one of the reasons for marriage is the 'procreation of children'. So for those for whom conception is a problem, the issues it raises are intensely personal but seldom private, and comments like 'When are you going to give me a grandchild?' from well-meaning in-laws can cut to the quick.

Not only will a couple have all this to deal with, there will also be the fear of the unknown and its outcome. Placing yourself under medical scrutiny is seldom pleasant, especially if you fear learning the worst. Time-consuming and often impersonal as medical tests are, they are a prerequisite to that medical goal, diagnosis, from which will come – it is hoped – a solution. For many couples this process, even if conception occurs relatively early on without recourse to the full-blown reproductive technology of IVF or other treatments, can test their relationship to the limits.

It is also a normal part of this process that some deeply buried resentments, anxieties and grief can be triggered and find expression in anger or the emotional isolation of a partner. Being aware of these possibilities can go some way to facing them head on and ensuring that the reasons why a couple wanted to be parents together do not become lost. This is not always easy to do without outside help, which explains why seeing a counsellor in order to talk through difficult feelings together can be enormously beneficial. There are also a number of support organisations which are well worth contacting. The professional counselling organisation, British Infertility Counselling Association, and the self-help group the Infertility Network (see Useful Addresses) can be enormously helpful in providing support and advice and practical suggestions.

In fact it is a legal requirement of the Human Fertilisation and Embryology Act that any clinic providing assisted conception – which may involve the use of donated eggs, sperm or embryos – must offer counselling to any patient or donor, in order that they can fully understand the individual and personal implications of their decisions. While this is specific to assisted conception, most clinics and others concerned with treating infertility recognise the emotional strain that can result from investigations and treatment and, as a consequence, would expect to offer some form of counselling to couples.

INVESTIGATIONS

One of the first tests carried out at the beginning of any infertility investigation is the previously mentioned semen analysis. Tests on women are more complex, time-consuming and ultimately expensive (whether done on the NHS or privately) so this relatively quick and easy test is usually the first done in order to rule out any immediate problem in the man while waiting to assess his partner. It is often a prerequisite of tests for a woman that her partner has had this done.

Even if sexual performance, ejaculation and the amount of semen produced all seem 'normal', it is only by microscopic examination of a fresh sample of semen that the quantity and quality of sperm produced can be assessed. Because sperm is being continually produced in the testes, and is therefore liable to vary depending on general health, exposure to environmental factors etc., two or more sperm counts are usually done at intervals to check over a period of time.

In order to examine a fresh semen sample under laboratory conditions a man usually has to produce this on-site, but although this is preferable some laboratories offer the option of producing it at home and bringing it in within two hours to the outpatients' clinic. This involves producing a sample by masturbation and collecting it in a container. Most men feel ambivalent about this procedure and some are afraid they will be unable to produce a sample. Staff in clinics are well aware of this anxiety and will do all they can to minimise embarrassment. However, compared to the infertility tests a woman may have to undergo, it remains a relatively uncomplicated, painless and non-invasive investigation and should be seen for what it is: an opportunity to try and solve a problem with conception.

Microscopic examination of semen will provide information not only about the quantity of sperm in the sample, but also the seminal fluid in which it is contained. If the sperm count is low, but the majority of the individual sperms are within the normal range, then it is likely that conception can occur eventually. About 70% of cases of male infertility are caused by a low sperm count. One of the reasons for testing more than one sperm count is to check whether sperm production is consistently low, or whether there is some variation as might be expected.

The yardstick against which semen analysis is measured covers the following:

- ◆ volume: this is usually around 2–5 ml. Too little volume and transportation becomes a problem, too much (over 5 ml. per ejaculate) and the sperm may be too heavily diluted to be effective;
- ◆ numbers of sperm; this should be 20 million plus per ml;
- ◆ motility: at least 40% of the sperm should be actively moving about;
- ◆ normality: at least 40% of the sperm should be normal in appearance.

However, if there are abnormalities in the sperm, or they are of poor motility (where they do not move properly) this may be for a number of reasons. There may be, for example, a sub-clinical infection that is affecting the quality of sperm production, or a problem with the man's hormonal levels. Sometimes a man may have a varicocele in the testes, a large vein similar to a varicose vein, which affects sperm production. In around 5% of infertile men, there are immunological problems affecting sperm production. Here, the man's body mistakenly identifies the sperm it produces as foreign, and it is attacked by his immune system, thus damaging it. Further investigations are necessary if the quality of the sperm proves to be poor, to identify the actual reason for this, and see if treatment is possible.

The results of this test should be given in person, and ideally to both partners at the same time. This may seem unnecessary if everything is fine, but if not it is appropriate that any less-than-welcome news is received by both partners together, that they should share in this and be there to support each other. It also reinforces the feeling that infertility is a joint problem, and consequently one to be tackled together.

Another test that may be used to examine sperm activity is the post-coital test, carried out on the woman. Many clinics no longer use this, partly because newer forms of effective treatment that by-pass the cervix have reduced its usefulness as a test procedure. However, it is a test that looks at how sperm functions once it is deposited within the woman's body, and can also give some indication of the effectiveness of the woman's cervical mucus secretions (which can also give a good indication of whether or not a woman is ovulating), and the general receptivity of the woman's body to her partner's sperm.

If carried out, this test needs to be done within six to thirty-six hours (the earlier the better) after sexual intercourse (coitus). The optimum time during the woman's fertility cycle for this test to be carried out is as close to ovulation as possible, when there should be an abundance of 'fertile-type' mucus, the very wet, stretchy mucus associated with ovulation, as described in chapter two, The Female fertility cycle. A sample of fluid is taken from the woman's cervix, in much the same way as a cervical smear is taken, and is immediately examined microscopically.

What the doctor hopes to see is a lot of normal and active sperm swimming around in receptive and easily-penetrated mucus. An apparently negative post-coital test can occur in normal couples for a number of reasons, and may need to be repeated. These reasons include the timing of the test with regard to the woman's cycle: too early or too late, and the cervical mucus would be less receptive or non-existent. It may be that during that month the woman has not ovulated, or on this occasion the quality of the man's sperm was poor.

More seriously, what this test might identify is a consistent problem in ovulation, especially if the test is done in the light of more general knowledge about the woman's cycle, perhaps because she has been charting her basal body temperature or cervical mucus symptoms. The test may also show that the man's sperm is again low in numbers, or abnormal in some way, following a sperm count test. It may be that there is some damage to the cervix, or some persistent infection. Or it may show that one or other partner is producing antibodies which are damaging the sperm.

Although the idea of making love and hot-footing it off to the outpatients clinic for this test may fill you with dismay, remember it can potentially clarify or identify certain key factors in the conception process that may or may not be occurring, and so it may be worthwhile. You may also think about requesting it if it is not offered, because of what it can tell you, thus helping you decide about further investigations or tests.

The full gamut of investigations offered to women to discern the cause of the problems they have in conceiving are specific to the area in which they may lie. As described above, the three main areas in which these may occur are concerned with the production of an egg and ovulation, the clear passage through the reproductive tract, and whether or not a fertilised egg successfully implants in the lining of the womb.

Tests to confirm if ovulation is occurring take a number of forms. An indication of this can be gleaned from temperature charting and cervical mucus secretions, as previously described. Ultrasound of the ovaries can also be done, as can blood or urine tests to check hormone levels to discover why ovulation may not be occurring.

There is also a saliva test available, but it is relatively new and may be difficult to obtain. The female hormone panel (FHP) is an extremely good way of evaluating a woman's hormonal balance during her cycle. Saliva samples are taken every other day, and require eleven samples to monitor the changing levels of oestrogen and progesterone. One study in 1989 (Finn, M.M. et al, Gynaecological Endocrinology) suggested that the saliva test gave a much more accurate picture of hormonal activity than did the previously mentioned progesterone blood test. From the information gained from the FHP test, it is possible to see whether a woman is ovulating, when in her cycle she is ovulating, whether there are any problems with the post-ovulation production of progesterone which is necessary for continuing pregnancy should fertilisation occur, and a number of other features relevant to conception. If you have a problem in finding out more about FHP testing, contact the Individual Wellbeing Diagnostic Laboratories (see Useful Addresses). Unfortunately the service is practitioner-only, so you can't self-refer, but you can get more information about the test to pass on to your doctor and ask him or her if it might be made available to you.

Your doctor might be more easily persuaded if you point out that it gives more information, and is more accurate, therefore more cost-effective than a blood test!

Internal examination of the female

A thorough internal examination, to check the position and normality of the uterus, whether there is any tenderness and where, and perhaps taking vaginal swabs to rule out infection, are all part of normal infertility investigations.

Ultrasound

Ultrasound can be done abdominally, but more frequently a vaginal ultrasound is done, which gives a more accurate picture of the ovaries and internal organs. For a vaginal ultrasound, the transducer or probe is lubricated and inserted in the vagina. One of the benefits of this is that it avoids the need for a full bladder so is more comfortable. With ultrasound done frequently during the time leading up to ovulation, it is possible to see the follicles maturing. When a follicle is about 20 mm in diameter, it suggests that ovulation is imminent.

Hysterosalpingogram

A special X-ray, called a hysterosalpingogram or HSG, taken of the womb and Fallopian tubes can very usefully indicate whether there are any abnormalities within the internal reproductive organs of a woman. This test needs to be done when there is no risk of pregnancy, and during the first half of the cycle before ovulation may have occurred is best. Radio-opaque dye, one that shows up on X-ray, is inserted into the womb via a very thin tube passed through the cervix. This fills the cavity of the womb and also travels into the Fallopian tubes. Any abnormality is clearly visible on screen, and a number of X-rays are taken. Any blockages may be a result of the tubes going into spasm and a laparoscopy may be needed to confirm a definite diagnosis of blocked tubes.

The whole procedure takes about ten minutes, does not require hospital admission and, for most women, is relatively painless. Any further discomfort is usually minimal, and since the introduction of less irritating radio-opaque dyes even this has been reduced.

Endometrial biopsy

Although this can be done alone, it is usually carried out as part of a laparoscopic investigation (see below).

Laparoscopy

A much more invasive, but very important test that is often carried out as part of infertility investigations is the laparoscopy. This involves a general anaesthetic and twenty-four hour hospital admission, although some centres now carry out laparoscopy as a day-care procedure. Laparoscopy enables the doctor to actually see inside the abdominal cavity, and look closely at the internal reproductive organs. A small incision is made near the navel, for the laparoscope itself and another near the pubic hairline that allows insertion of a probe. In order to get a clearer look at things, a small amount of carbon dioxide is used to inflate the abdominal cavity a little and allow easier movement of both the laparoscope and the probe.

Not only can the doctor see very clearly whether there are any abdominal adhesions, any evidence of endometriosis, or abnormalities of the body of the womb, if the procedure is carried out after ovulation it is possible to see that this has occurred by looking at the ovaries. In addition, a coloured fluid can be inserted via the cervix to see if it runs through the Fallopian tubes, which can indicate whether or not there is a blockage within these. If this is done, it is often referred to as a 'lap and dye': medical shorthand for laparoscopy and dye. The laparoscope also has the facility for taking internal photographs which are of surprisingly good quality and may be interesting for you to see. For many women, the up-side of this physically and emotionally demanding procedure will be that it reassures them that, even if everything is not perfect internally, the problem is diagnosed and a solution may be possible.

A laparoscopy, used just for diagnostic purposes, usually takes around thirty minutes to complete. Sometimes it is possible for the doctor to carry out surgical procedures using this opportunity, perhaps to remove small areas of endometriosis using diathermy or laser to, literally, burn them off. Occasionally more complex procedures, perhaps to open the blocked end of one of the Fallopian tubes, can be undertaken in this way but it depends on the skill and inclination of the surgeon. Surgical procedures undertaken during laparoscopy extend the time of the operation.

Although it is not necessary to have a general anaesthetic to have an endometrial biopsy done, it is sometimes done during the laparoscopic procedure. Inserting a thin instrument in order to scrape a sample from the lining of the womb, the endometrium, via the cervix can cause period-like cramping for some women who may prefer to be under anaesthetic when it is done. An endometrial biopsy really needs to be done during the second half of a woman's cycle though, because if ovulation has occurred then this will be indicated by the effect of the progesterone, secreted by the post-ovulation corpus luteum, on the lining of the womb.

Following laparoscopy, many women experience some post-anaesthetic wooziness while others may feel sick. In addition, referred pain in the shoulders, caused by the carbon dioxide used to inflate the abdominal cavity irritating the nerves of the abdominal lining, can cause discomfort for some for a day or two. But post-operative pain should be virtually non-existent because the sites of entry, usually two incisions at the navel and pubic hairline, are so small. These are usually sutured with a dissolvable stitch which is best kept dry for the first twenty-four to forty-eight hours.

The main investigative procedures are outlined above, but there are a number of 'optional' tests which may or may not be available to you either because of resources, or because they are unnecessary: those already carried out have been enough to present a diagnostic picture. These may include blood hormone profiles for both men and women, which might include a look at prolactin or thyroid hormone levels in a woman, or testosterone levels in a man.

Whatever other tests are recommended, there will be reasons for these that are quite specific to you and as a consequence need to be discussed fully with your infertility specialist. However, for the majority of couples, the progress of infertility investigations proceeds or ceases based on what is discovered at each stage. It would be unusual for a couple to have test after test after test without discerning some clue as to why conception was problematic. What is important is not to allow testing to drag on for an extended length of time, but to make quite clear decisions at each stage, based on individual circumstances. For example, a couple in their twenties where the woman seems to be functioning normally but the man has a low sperm count, may want to carry on unassisted *because they have the time and opportunity to do so*. But this situation immediately changes if this same couple were in their late thirties, where the woman's natural ability to conceive may be declining.

What becomes apparent from this is the way in which a couples' problems with conceiving are so unique to them and their joint circumstances. This is why the relationship with their doctor, and their ability to understand enough about what is happening in order to make decisions pertinent to their own lives, is so important.

'Although I was happy to go ahead with further investigations when we discovered that Josie wasn't ovulating regularly, I don't think it was as important for me as it was for her. I think we were very lucky that she conceived – without intervention – when she did. I'm not sure I would have been very happy to go through IVF if it had come to that.'

Gareth, aged 32

'I thought children would just be a nice optional extra in our marriage, until the doctor said that Michael's semen analysis showed that his sperm production was a bit on the low side. We weren't ever sure that this was the whole reason why we hadn't conceived after two years, but because we were still in our twenties, I wasn't too bothered. Until the doctor said that Michael's sperm might be a problem. Then I thought, help, this is what I've always wanted! And then we really gave it our best shot. We had more sex during that six months than ever before — and it seemed to work! Anyway, I got pregnant and he's now two and I'm pregnant again.'

Caro, aged 28

6 Treatments for infertility

'It was such a relief to have my "problem" diagnosed. Now, at least, I felt as if we knew what we were up against. What I had found so difficult before was just not knowing. Although I knew we had a long way to go, it was just so much better than not knowing.'

Kath, aged 33

'Twelve years ago, I found myself unable to conceive at thirty-five, and was referred for treatment by my doctor. Much is written about infertility, but unless you're infertile and denied a woman's basic need to conceive, it's impossible to imagine the pain and sense of uselessness. After a year of treatment which seemed unending – blood tests, investigative surgery, scans and injections – I became pregnant and gave birth to a beautiful boy.'

Jenny, now 47

Any treatment offered to correct or improve a problem that is making conception difficult will be based on a diagnosis made following any tests or investigations carried out. Treatments described in this chapter are designed to help a couple conceive on their own, and are different from reproductive technologies that assist conception, which are covered in a later chapter.

Perhaps the simplest way to review what treatments for difficulties in conception might be available, or offered, is to look at the reasons behind them. The reasons for which treatment might be offered in the first place. Only medical treatments are outlined below, alternative and complementary approaches are covered in a separate chapter, but they may well be worth consideration if you are wanting to make a comprehensive assessment of what is on offer, and what is right for you.

FAILURE TO OVULATE

Clomiphene

If tests have shown that a woman is not ovulating, or ovulates haphazardly, then it is possible to prescribe drug treatment that will stimulate ovulation. The first drug of choice is usually Clomiphene, or Clomid, and should only be prescribed by a fertility specialist and only when a complete diagnosis of ovulation problems has been made. Be wary if your GP prescribes it without ensuring that other reasons behind an apparent failure to conceive have been ruled out. One woman was prescribed it by her GP, even though it was her husband's low sperm count that was thought to be the problem. She was sure, from charting her temperature over several months, that she was ovulating. After a while, having tolerated various minor side-effects of the drug, it occurred to her that there was probably no necessity for *her* to be taking it, given that the problem lay with her husband! The GP's view had been that it might be worthwhile, just in case ovulation was not already occurring, but he had not really checked.

The downside of Clomiphene is that it affects cervical mucus, thickening it and making it less accessible to the transportation of sperm. In some cases it may also make the lining of the womb less available to a fertilised egg for implantation. Neither of which will assist conception. Occasionally the ovaries can react to this drug negatively and become cystic. So careful monitoring, perhaps with ultrasound and blood tests, are often recommended while treatment with Clomiphene continues.

The success rate with Clomiphene is only around 50%, even

though around 80% of women achieve regular ovulation through its use. For some women, conception occurs after she has ceased taking the drug, as if there is some sort of rebound effect. Side effects of the drug can include mood swings, headaches, and occasionally pelvic pains if the ovaries become swollen in response to Clomiphene – a 14% risk. There is also an increased risk of multiple pregnancy, around one in twenty.

'Although I was warned that I might experience some "mood swings" while taking Clomiphene, I think this was an understatement! What I actually experienced was amazing bursts of irritability – bordering on real rage – over really quite inconsequential things. I managed to keep a lid on it at work, but my partner really got the brunt of it. If we hadn't been so committed to trying for a baby, I'm not sure I could have put up with it.'

Carrie, aged 31

'Apart from feeling a little nauseous occasionally, I didn't really notice much of a reaction. In fact, after all the dire warnings about side effects, I wasn't particularly convinced that it was working.

Rose, aged 29

Bromocriptine

If a diagnosis has been made of increased prolactin production by the pituitary gland, which is inhibiting ovulation, then this drug can be highly effective. Raised prolactin levels are an uncommon cause of infertility, but if they exist, this is the treatment usually offered.

Very occasionally, this raised prolactin level is because of a benign pituitary tumour, which may also be affecting levels of other pituitary hormones. Treating this with bromocriptine is often all that is required, but if the tumour is large enough to cause problems elsewhere because of its size, perhaps affecting the eyesight, then surgical removal is usually advised.

Human chorionic gonadotrophin (HCG)

Given by injection, this is similar in effect to luteinising hormone (LH) which stimulates the ovarian follicle to release a mature egg (ovulation). It is often given to a woman who is already being treated with Clomiphene, designed to stimulate the follicle to produce an egg. However, the timing of these injections is important, in order to work in close conjunction with the useful effects of the Clomiphene, so ultrasound and blood tests may also be necessary to monitor progress.

Human menopausal gonadotrophin (HMG)

Surprising though it may seem, menopausal women produce increased quantities of follicle stimulating hormone (FSH) and luteinising hormone in a last-ditch attempt to stimulate ovarian activity. These two hormones are excreted in the urine of menopausal women, and from this is HMG produced, usually referred to by brand names Pergonal or Humegon.

Its most useful and active component is the FSH and it can be highly effective. But it is a powerful drug, given by injection during the first part of a woman's cycle, and in combination with an injection of HCG in order to ensure that the release of an egg – ovulation – is stimulated.

Its most common useage is, in fact, as a preliminary to IVF where the ability to stimulate the ovary to produce more than one egg follicle at a time, is useful in the collection of several eggs for fertilisation. This use is covered more comprehensively in the chapter on assisted conception.

It is a drug that does require careful monitoring. Some women, and it is not possible to tell beforehand which may be susceptible, find that their ovaries become hyperstimulated through its use. They can become enlarged, cystic and painful. In addition, because it is not possible to gauge the overall effect of the drug on individual women, then the stimulation of the development of more than one follicle, and the release of one or more eggs at ovulation, increases the risk of multiple pregnancy, which is not without its own risk to both the mother and her unborn babies.

It is also an expensive drug to administer, which has some bearing on its availability. Because of both its need for careful monitoring of a woman receiving this drug, and its cost, it is often only given for a three-month period, after which its use in a particular patient's treatment is reviewed.

Buserelin

It is not always clear at first why a drug that actually suppresses the function of the pituitary gland can help with infertility. Buserelin is a short-acting drug, taken as a nasal spray every four hours. It makes production of FSH and LH by the pituitary gland fall, after an initial burst of activity. Once the levels of these two hormones are low, then a woman's ovaries cease activity and no longer produce oestrogen.

It is most used as a preliminary to giving HMG, described above, because the combined effect of giving buserelin and then HMG is that the ovaries are stimulated more effectively. In addition, the ovary is often stimulated so effectively it will produce more than one egg at a time. This is why the use of these two drugs most often occurs prior to IVF treatment (see chapter seven, Assisted conception).

Again, these drugs are usually only given under close supervision in a specialist unit. Their effects are potentially powerful, and most women taking them experienced a range of symptoms as a result. Headaches, night sweats and mood changes are among those tolerated by many women.

Danazol

This is a drug used to help alleviate the symptoms of endometriosis, although its use does in fact stop ovulation. Endometriosis can be a chronic and debilitating gynaecological disorder in some women. Patches of endometrial tissue appear around a woman's internal organs, other than in its normal place in the lining of the womb, and respond to the normal cycle of hormonal changes that occur in the lining of the womb. This means that as the endometrium thickens and is then shed, patches of endometrial tissue appearing perhaps in the Fallopian tubes, or on the ovaries, are doing the same. This continued process can lead to pain, infections, blockages and adhesions. It is a very difficult diagnosis to come to terms with.

Ironically, if a diagnosis of endometriosis is made in a young woman, the recommended advice is to 'get pregnant' because the pregnancy itself reduces many of the symptoms of endometriosis. The other reason for this emphasis is that, the longer a woman suffers endometriosis, the greater the likelihood that it will damage her chances of conceiving at a later date. So, many young women are presented with something of a dilemma if a well-meaning, but perhaps a little thoughtless, suggestion like this is made.

'I couldn't believe it when the doctor said the best thing was to have a baby. I was twenty-two and had just left university. Although I had a boyfriend, we weren't at the stage of our relationship where having children was anything like on the agenda! I wasn't ready to settle down yet either. There was so much I wanted to do and I had never thought there would be this sort of pressure on me about children, so early.'

Nicky, aged 33

'It was a real dilemma. I wasn't ready to become a mother, but should I wait and risk infertility at thirty? I took a risk, and was treated on and off with Danazol during the intervening years. I just thought that, surely things would improve, and I did try to stay fit and healthy. I did conceive after nearly a year of trying, and I don't know for sure whether my endometriosis made any difference to the time it took because I was still, as the doctors said, within the normal range for my age. Getting pregnant the second time, eighteen months after the first, was quicker.'

Lissa, aged 37

Certainly an Australian study on endometriosis showed that among women with endometriosis who managed to become pregnant, 40% had no further problems. But in the remaining 60%, symptoms returned within a one- to four-year period. So for some women, pregnancy is not the hormonal cure it might be.

Danazol is hormonally similar to the male hormone testosterone, so is effective in preventing ovulation and stopping the menstrual cycle, and shrinking the endometrium, wherever it appears. However, taking it is not always without problems. Many women experience weight gain and tiredness, especially at first. Other symptoms also include nausea, depression, hot flushes, acne, loss of libido, increased body hair and a deepening of the voice. Not everyone will experience any, or all, of these symptoms but if side effects occur, then there may be other alternatives which suit you better and your doctor can advise you.

Other hormonal treatment includes taking the contraceptive pill for an extended period, with no breaks, to reduce the activity of the endometrium and allow things to settle down. Progestogens, usually Duphaston or Primolet N, may also be prescribed because they inhibit menstrual bleeding and help shrink areas of endometriosis. These can sometimes be used if Danazol is producing unwanted or unpleasant side effects.

While effective in treating the symptoms of endometriosis, these hormonal treatments make conception impossible because they inhibit the normal hormonal function of the woman's fertility cycle. They may be helpful in the long run though, because following treatment conception becomes possible as inflammation, residual swelling and subsequent blockages are reduced.

The severity of endometriosis symptoms varies enormously from woman to woman. Some women have few symptoms, but a severe problem with conceiving. Others have quite pronounced areas of endometriosis, but it does not prevent conception. It is often to do with where the patches of endometriosis occur. If inflammation and scarring of both tubes results, then conception may be impossible, and surgical treatment may be the only option.

SURGICAL TREATMENTS

Endometriosis

Surgical treatment, or laser treatment, can be successful in reducing areas of endometriosis and scar tissue. Success depends in part on where the patches of endometriosis may be. If the damage is to the very delicate Fallopian tubes, it may not be possible to reconstruct the tubes adequately enough to promote conception and the only option may be assisted conception with IVF.

'After surgery I was put on Danazol which had severe side effects, so my doctors suggested Duphaston instead. I kept getting breakthrough bleeding, even when I went up to the highest dose. I gave up and changed to Primolut N. Nine months' treatment did the trick, and I have been free of symptoms for the past five years.'

Dina, aged 29

The National Endometriosis Society (see Useful Addresses) is a charitable self-help support and information group who will be able to provide up-to-date information about treatment and its availability.

Polycystic ovaries

It is not really known why polycystic ovarian syndrome occurs, but it is primarily the result of excessive hormonal activity, where the ovaries are over-stimulated and attempt to produce too many follicles. These fluid-filled cavities make the ovary swell and give it a cystic appearance – it looks covered with cysts. The cysts create a toughening of the ovarian capsule making follicle development and ovulation difficult in some women. It is a very common occurrence and it is thought that perhaps as many as one woman in five or six has some sort of problem.

Surgically removing a section of the ovary used to be the treatment offered, because this seemed to allow the ovary to function better, and in some cases it was particularly effective. This is done less often today, and has been more or less replaced by the use of laparoscopic or microscopic surgical techniques instead. This allows surgeons the opportunity to make a small diathermic incision to the ovary, with good therapeutic effect and less risk of complications from more invasive surgery that sometimes can arise.

Polycystic ovarian syndrome, despite being a relatively common problem, is poorly understood. In some women it causes little or no problem with conception, whereas in others it may create great difficulties. Specialists have different approaches to this problem, although the only real treatment available is as described above. Diagnosis with ultrasound is relatively straightforward, and it may be suspected as a cause of infertility if a woman also experiences symptoms of weight gain and excessive hair growth, particularly on the face. But it is just as usual to have no associated symptoms.

'At the very first ultrasound, the doctor said to me, 'Oh, you've got polycystic ovaries, that's your problem.' I was taken aback because I didn't know about polycystic ovaries then. There were no signs early on. There was a long period when I felt betrayed and alienated by my body. I would look at my belly and think what the hell's going on in there, why doesn't it work?

Miranda, aged 32

Fibroids

These benign growths develop from the myometrium, the middle layer of the lining of the womb. Some fibroids are completely contained within the wall of the womb, some protrude into the cavity of the womb and some protrude through the external wall of the womb into the pelvic cavity, and they sometimes cause problems with conception. Depending on their size, and where in the womb they occur, fibroids or polyps could inhibit the implantation of a fertilised egg, or even its smooth descent from Fallopian tube to womb, because it is blocking this opening.

Fibroids are relatively common; it is thought that around one in five women have them to some degree. They are more common in women who have never been pregnant, in older women and in women of Afro-Caribbean origin. Many women have them and they cause no problem at all, but during infertility investigations they may show up and may need surgical removal.

Sometimes fibroids are felt during a routine internal examination, or they show up on ultrasound, especially vaginal ultrasound. A standard abdominal X-ray may show them quite clearly, or during internal laproscopic examination. However they are diagnosed, they are relatively easy to remove surgically, although the proof that they are a direct cause of failure to conceive will only be evident if pregnancy occurs. In other words, although well worth removing, fibroids and polyps may not have been the definitive reason for failure to conceive.

Polyps

Polyps can be removed quite simply during a D&C (dilatation and curettage), often referred to more colloquially as a 'scrape', which more or less describes what happens. Large polyps may need surgical removal. As with fibroids, many women with polyps have no trouble conceiving but they may be worth removing in women who do.

Blockages and adhesions

Microsurgery has greatly improved surgical repair of damage to the Fallopian tubes. Pelvic infections that produced scarring, resulting in blockages that created problems with conception, now have an increased chance of successful repair. This success is also dependent on a number of factors including extent of the damage and where it occurs. For example, if tubes are blocked at the opening into the womb, there is greater success than if they are blocked at the outer end, where the fimbria meet the ovaries. So the success rates can vary as widely as between 30% to 65% and part of this is also dependent on the skill and expertise of the surgeon carrying out the procedure.

Where damage is diagnosed by laparoscopic examination, and shown to be too extensive to warrant an attempt at repair, the advice may only leave assisted conception – IVF – as an option. There is also some evidence to suggest that any surgical interference with the Fallopian tubes increases the risk of further infection, although this is greatly minimised with microscopic surgical techniques, and also the risk of ectopic pregnancy.

Congenital abnormalities

Some women are born with an abnormally shaped womb, which can give rise to problems with conception, but this is a rare occurrence. The three main abnormalities are a septate uterus, where the womb has a septum that separates the internal cavity into two halves; a double uterus where there are, effectively two wombs joined together; and a rudimentary uterine horn, which is generally considered to be similar to a double uterus with one less well developed than the other.

These conditions are unusual, but are a relatively easy-to-diagnose cause of infertility. With a septate uterus in particular, the egg is often successfully fertilised but problems with implantation cause repeated miscarriage. Surgical correction of these abnormalities can be successful, with a 65% to 75% chance of pregnancy.

Reversal of sterilisation

Any woman requesting sterilisation, or tubal ligation, for contraceptive purposes should be fully advised that this is considered an irreversible operation. Sterilisation is usually only recommended after a woman has completed her family, because the possibility of reversal of sterilisation is so remote. However, because of the advances in micro-surgery in recent years, there is a greater possibility of successful reversal, if it is possible to find a surgeon with the appropriate expertise (this may only be available privately). Alternatively, the other option if reversal is unsuccessful is assisted conception through IVF but again, this might not be available on the NHS under these circumstances.

INFECTIONS

While past infections within the female reproductive organs can give rise to problems with blockages and adhesions, and cause infertility as we have seen, other low-grade but persistent infections can create problems with conception for a number of reasons. Infections can create a hostile internal environment for sperm, as well as create problems with implantation. Some doctors think that infections like chlamydia which often have no discernible symptoms, and go un-diagnosed, can reduce a couple's chances of conception.

'I had no idea I had any sort of infection, and I was mortified when I was referred to the STD clinic for tests, even though it was explained to me that this was purely because they have the best facilities and resources for testing on the spot. I had chlamydia, which cleared after treatment with antibiotics – but I had had no symptoms, so had no way of knowing. My partner was treated to just to ensure he had no infection he could pass back to me. I was relieved that it was so easy to treat, and that our doctor had thought to get it checked out.'

Debbie, aged 29

This may well be why a GP recommends that a woman is tested for infection and, possibly, her partner too. Taking swabs to culture may not be effective at isolating an infection. Looking immediately at a vaginal swab sample under a microscope may be more helpful, but demands the facilities and expertise to do so and for this you might find yourself referred to a genito-urinary (GU) or sexually-transmitted diseases (STD) clinic. This is only because they have facilities for immediate analysis to hand, not because your doctor thinks that you have some sort of sinister disease.

Other doctors may give you a broad-spectrum antibiotic in the hope that this will kill off any residual bacterial infection. Accurate diagnosis and analysis of bacterial sensitivity to a particular antibiotic means treatment is likely to be more conclusive. In any event, if you are prescribed any course of antibiotics, make sure you follow the instructions about dosage and timing and be sure you *complete the course*. If for any reason you react unfavourably to the antibiotics prescribed, do not just stop taking them without returning to your doctor for advice. It is often possible to prescribe an alternative. In most cases of infection, treatment is highly effective. So be reassured!

MEN

The main cause of male infertility is low, or absent, sperm count or sperm of poor quality or motility. This accounts for about 70% of male infertility, and can occur for a variety of reasons. Any treatment that may be possible will depend on its cause. Very few men are infertile, only around 5% produce no sperm at all. It is difficult to find a cause for total failure to produce sperm, which makes it equally difficult to treat.

If the cause of reduced sperm production is thought to be hormonal, there is also very little that can be done to improve it. Although a number of hormone replacement drugs are often tried, including testosterone, mesterolone and others, the final outcome seems to be poor in most cases, with little improvement in sperm production.

Very few men are able to accept the diagnosis of a low sperm count with equanimity. While any reason for difficulties in conception can be hard to take on board for either partner, a deficit in sperm production or quality seems to strike at the heart of a man's feelings about his masculinity. For this reason many men become quite distressed and depressed at such a diagnosis. Fear of such a diagnosis may also make many men reluctant to face the tests necessary to rule out problems in this area, as well as identifying such a problem, or its extent, prior to finding treatment.

'I couldn't believe it when I was told that the semen analysis showed such a low sperm count. Even when I was told that conception at this level was still possible, I felt somehow deficient, as if I'd let Paula down.'

Steve, aged 27

'I'd had children with my first wife, so I had assumed that the 'problem' with getting pregnant lay with Cherry. But it turned out that, although she had some inflammation in the left Fallopian tube, and only ovulated haphazardly, my sperm count was really quite low. We were told that, in spite of this combination of circumstances, there was no reason why we shouldn't be successful in the end. Still, I can't say it wasn't a shock.'

Tom, aged 42

'My sperm count was so low that the doctors advised IVF straightaway. Because Liz was thirty-three they didn't feel we should hang about, partly because the policy of no IVF on the NHS after thirty-five operates in our health trust.'

Doug, aged 38

Because of the continual nature of sperm production, it is susceptible to general fluctuations in health and external influences. Drinking alcohol in excess, smoking heavily and using marijuana are all known to influence sperm production. Overheating of the testicles is now considered to be less responsible for reduced sperm counts than was previously thought. The old idea about cold baths, and splashing ice-cold water on the testicles is now thought to be pretty useless, unless perhaps as some interesting new style of sexual foreplay.

Recent press reports about the global fall in sperm counts, linking it to various forms of environmental and chemical pollution, show no evidence, as yet, of this affecting conception rates overall. Most men continue to have a sperm analysis well within the normal range. While we are right to be concerned about environmental pollutants, and our own misuse of global resources, this needs to be kept in perspective with regard to infertility issues. A man's general health is much more important to sperm production than the possible environmental hazards that may exist.

Varicocele

A varicocele is a vein in the testicle that has become enlarged or distended in some way, and become varicosed or swollen. This can cause pressure, depending on its position, size, etc. on the tiny tubules through which the developing sperm have to pass. Around 20% of fertile men also have this condition, so while it is worth correcting in an apparently infertile man it still may not be the complete reason for a couple's inability to conceive successfully.

Treatment is simple, quick and relatively pain-free, involving an overnight hospital stay at most. If the varicocele is treated using a chemical injection to block the offending vein, thus reducing the possibility of swelling, then a local anaesthetic is probably all that is required.

Blocked tubes

Occasionally the tiny tubes of the testes, the epididymis and vas deferens, through which sperm have to travel prior to ejaculation, become blocked. Advances in microsurgery have increased the possibilities of unblocking these. If the tubes have been blocked for some time, sperm production will eventually have ceased and even after successfully unblocking these tubes, it may not mean the man is fertile again. The success of this surgery, (between 20% to 30% of men with a blocked tube will produce normal sperm afterwards) is very largely dependent on the skill of the surgeon as it is technically very difficult.

Infection

The presence of some sort of bacterial infection in the genital tract of the man can have an impact on sperm production, and on both its quantity and quality. For example, the difficult-to-diagnose chlamydia can cause epididymitis (inflammation of the epididymis). Checking this out, isolating any infection and treating it accordingly, can dramatically improve matters. The benefits of a course of antibiotics in clearing any infection will not show an immediate improvement in sperm production as this takes between four to six weeks.

Reversal of vasectomy

Men who have opted for vasectomy as an irreversible form of contraception, sometimes wish to increase their family later, perhaps because they now have a new partner with whom they wish to have children. Again, counselling at the time of opting for this minor operation should have made it clear how very difficult it is to reverse the effects of the original surgery. However, using micro-surgery techniques, it may be possible to attempt a reversal even if the success of the outcome cannot be guaranteed.

Even if there is limited sperm, or none at all, in the ejaculate following reversal of a vasectomy, it may be possible to use a new technique called PESA (Percutaneous Epididymal Sperm Aspiration) or TESE (Testicular Sperm Extraction) in conjunction with ICSI (Intra-Cytoplasmic Sperm Injection) to achieve conception (see page 113). Where there are persistent problems with the quality and quantity of the sperm, then there are a number of methods of assisted conception that improve the possibilities for successful conception in these cases. These are covered in a separate chapter.

7 Alternative and complementary therapies

'I really started seeing the homeopath because my mum thought it would help my feelings of anxiety while I was waiting for the hospital referral. The first thing I found so useful was the time she took to talk through everything with me. I know now that because the approach is holistic this is an important part of it, especially when it comes to prescribing a constitutional remedy, but it was equally useful as a way to try and work out exactly how I was feeling about a possible diagnosis of infertility.'

Kay, aged 27

'Seeing an acupuncturist was something I had done off and on for years, because I tend to get cluster headaches when I'm under stress. When the doctor said he thought I might have had an ectopic pregnancy, and that there may have been some inflammation in one of my tubes, I was off for some acupuncture like a shot. I just knew that it would help revitalise and heal me, and I felt I must try it before I got on to some sort of reproductive technology rollercoaster.'

Helen, aged 31

More and more people are using alternative and complementary therapies for a wide variety of conditions and ailments, and as part of a more holistic approach to the prevention and treatment of disease. Britons spend £130 million a year on complementary treatments and it is estimated that this will exceed more than £200 million by 2012 according to research published in 2008 by the Prince of Wales' Foundation for Integrated Health (www.fihealth.org.uk), which also estimated that such therapies were being used regularly by around six million people a year. Greater efforts to regulate the CAM industry have resulted in better availability, but it still remains on the fringe of modern medicine, unable to secure the research funding that might conclusively prove or disprove its efficacy. However, because of continued public interest and use, the NHS Trusts' Association has responded by publishing a useful directory of complementary and alternative practitioners, available to download from their website www.nhsta.org.uk

The most popular therapies are, in descending order, homeopathy, osteopathy, acupuncture and aromatherapy. While the majority of therapists have to be consulted privately, more and more doctors and nurses are extending their professional practice by qualifying in one or more complementary health therapies, and you may find that you have a practitioner among the staff available to you at your local health centre. What is clearly important is that whoever you consult is properly qualified and registered. To check this out, look for registration credentials or consult the recognised authoritative bodies if necessary (see Useful Addresses).

This is especially important if you choose to consult an alternative practitioner in order to complement any treatment you may be having for problems in conceiving. Both the potential and efficacy of alternative therapies have to be balanced against their limitations. Understanding this means that you know what benefits may be gained specific to you, without creating unrealistic expectations. You cannot, for instance, expect acupuncture to unblock your tubes, but if you are having IVF, then it may help you in strengthening your system and preparing for that.

You may want to consider some form of alternative therapy in order to prepare for pregnancy, so enhancing your general health, or because you have a known problem, or because there seems to be no apparent reason why you are unable to conceive. Whatever your reasons, a full discussion with a qualified practitioner will identify your particular needs and any treatment will be on this basis. Because the emphasis is on helping the body to help itself, practitioners seldom talk in terms of a cure. They may also give you advice about your general health, and recommend changes to diet or lifestyle that are also beneficial. And recommendations about an additional source of alternative help may also be made, for example a homeopath may recommend a short course of acupuncture or vice versa.

While the general acceptance of alternative therapies increases daily, and also the recognition of their value as an additional resource in treatment, there is little other than anecdotal evidence to confirm or deny their claims. In addition, many of us conversant with a Westernised approach to medicine – make a diagnosis, find a cure – find the more holistic approach difficult to accommodate intellectually. Many people find the idea of energy channels, to which numerous alternative therapies refer, difficult to understand although we readily accept the small amounts of electrical energy that occur at every nerve synapse, and the electrical energy that keeps our hearts beating. And while the idea of 'memories' of physical and emotional trauma being locked into our muscles is often derided, we readily accept the continued reproduction of scar tissue and new skin cells continuously repeating the trauma to the body of the original cut. The mind, body, spirit connection leaves many sceptics cold but no matter, you do not have to *believe* in alternative therapies for them to work. Keep an open mind, and find out what you can because as a resource in a multi-faceted approach to dealing with a problem, they have much to recommend them. The purpose of this chapter is to outline the main therapies you may wish to consider, even if you eventually reach the conclusion that they are not for you.

What is paramount is finding a practitioner you like and trust, because their help may be invaluable if you find yourself continuing to have problems with conception. And, if you find yourself going down the route of assisted conception, which can be both physically demanding and emotionally stressful, then the therapeutic back-up of your alternative practitioner, in whichever discipline, can be immensely supportive.

HOMEOPATHY

The principle of homeopathy is that 'like cures like', which is rather simplistic. In reality a tiny dose of a substance that creates similar symptoms will stimulate the body's own self-healing mechanism. For example, one remedy for itchy rashes is Rhus. Tox which is derived from poison ivy, a plant notorious for causing an itchy rash. Through its use, Rhus. Tox will stimulate the body's own resources to deal with a rash and cure itself.

Homeopathy can be used to treat symptoms, but it also has a constitutional role to play, and can treat the whole person, which is where the skill and expertise of the practitioner comes in. So while one remedy might be recommended for stimulating the pituitary gland, or for use where there have been recurrent miscarriages, an additional remedy might be prescribed to balance your overall constitution. This explains some of the apparently odd questions asked about seemingly unrelated subjects, for example whether you feel better on a windy day, or whether you sigh a lot. Used constitutionally, homeopathy enhances and improves general health.

It wasn't a question of either/or for me, it just made sense to try and regularise my periods when I wanted to try for a baby. They had always been a bit difficult and irregular, and I suppose I harboured this fear that it was somehow related to my fertility. This wasn't the sort of thing my GP would have considered a problem, although I'm sure he would have been sympathetic. I mean, the usual approach to difficult or irregular periods is to prescribe the pill! A friend recommended homeopathy, so I thought it worth a try.

'First I had a long and detailed consultation, including questions that made no sense to me! Then I was given a single dose of Nux Vomica x200, with a less potent dosage subsequently. In addition I was given

sulphur, and after several months the constitutional remedy Calcarea Carbonicum. I must stress that what was prescribed for me was what was right for me, and no one else. And it worked. My periods regularised and were much less troublesome, so I suppose my whole reproductive system was responding positively. Certainly conception wasn't a problem, and I was pregnant around seven months after I started taking the homeopathic remedies prescribed for me.'

Lindy, aged 27

One aspect of homeopathy many people find difficult to accept is the greater the dilution of the remedy, the greater its potency. For example, a remedy marked x6 has been diluted six times, while x30 has been diluted thirty times. However the more potent remedy is the x30. Generally, the lower potency dose is used for symptomatic treatment, while the higher potency dose is used in emergencies, or in treating chronic conditions.

Remedies are taken by mouth, preferably in between meals and without strong substances – coffee, toothpaste, tobacco, for example – still in evidence, which will antidote the remedy and render it ineffectual. If necessary the mouth should be thoroughly rinsed with clear water. Remedies should not be touched other than by the person for whom they are intended, and then only minimally. Remedies come in a variety of forms – pills, tablets, granules, for example – and should be transferred from container to the mouth on a clean spoon.

An initial consultation usually lasts around an hour, while subsequent visits will be shorter. Average costs can range from between £40 and £75 and some private health schemes will cover the cost of homeopathic treatment. You can expect to need a series of appointments, with follow-ups after the initial consultation, especially if the problem is long-standing.

Some doctors are also registered homeopaths and they may be able to prescribe remedies on the NHS, although a prescription charge is likely to be more expensive than the direct cost from a supplier. Details of the authorised bodies for homeopaths, and mail order suppliers and the other alternative therapists in this chapter, can be found in the back of the book (see Useful Addresses).

OSTEOPATHY

Osteopathy is well-known as a treatment for problems with the spine but, more holistically, it can have an impact on the whole body. Correcting musculo-skeletal problems also has a positive effect on both blood flow and the lymphatic system when tension is released. Osteopathic practitioners who also have training in cranial therapy work less with high-velocity thrusts, for which osteopathy is known, but with a very gentle and specific focus on the spine and cranial bones of the skull. This cranio-sacral work is no less dynamic, and has an impact on the subtle fluctuations of the cerebro-spinal fluid, easing any blockages in the flow and rebalancing the body.

Osteopathy is not confined to manipulation of bones as its techniques are also applied to ligaments, muscles and internal organs. And correcting musculo-skeletal problems can have a direct effect on internal organs. For example, a problem with an upper cervical vertebrae in the neck could cause tension in the pituitary gland. Easing this problem may improve the function of the pituitary gland, which would have a positive impact on hormone production. In addition, a lower back problem may create tension in the internal reproductive organs, so easing this might improve matters there. Certainly there has been anecdotal evidence to suggest this to be the case in patients with unexplained infertility who, following treatment with osteopathy and cranial osteopathy, have gone on to conceive successfully.

'I had always seen an osteopath, on and off for years, with an occasional back problem. I felt she knew my body very well so when we were having some sort of delay in conceiving, and hospital tests showed I had a hydrosalpinx [fluid and swelling in the Fallopian tube], I went to see her to talk it through and ask her advice.

'She did a lot of work around my lower back, working to free things up and to help the general drainage in this area, as well as doing a bit of an overhaul in preparation for pregnancy. What also really helped was her belief that improvements could be made, and that conception would be possible. This very holistic approach really helped my confidence, and whether this influenced my chances or not, I did conceive.'

Helen, aged 34

Osteopathy is not something that can provide a one-off cure, so expect to have at least a series of visits. If there is an acute problem, then a visit to treat that alone might be a one-off, but usually only in the context of a longer association as a practitioner gets to know you and your body and can begin to treat you more holistically. Costs can vary between £50 to £75 for a first consultation, and then subsequent visits may be anything between £45 to £70. Some doctors will be happy to refer you for treatment under the NHS, but this is not always possible. And many health insurance policies will cover osteopathic treatment, although not always for chronic problems.

Again, because of the holistic approach in treatment provided by osteopathic practitioners, many individuals have found this therapy beneficial not only for a specific problem but also for their general health. Finding a registered practitioner, if not through personal recommendation, is possible through their official registration body.

ACUPUNCTURE

Acupuncture forms part of traditional Chinese medicine, and is becoming more and more accepted in the West, partly because so many people find it effective for a variety of complaints. It works on the principle that our individual health is maintained by an internal energy flow along specific channels, or meridians, within the body. This energy flow is referred to as Qi (pronounced chee) and should this be blocked or interrupted, then an imbalance occurs between the two energy forces of the body, described as Yin and Yang. Yin represents traditional feminine qualities of softness and calm, while Yang represents traditional masculine qualities of stimulation and aggression

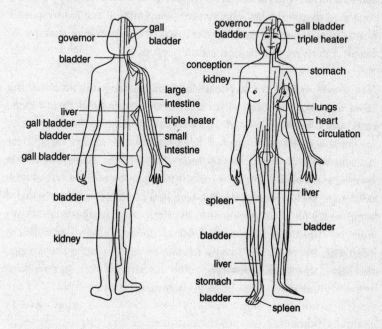

Acupuncture meridian points

There are twelve main energy channels, connected to and named after an internal organ. There are also eight extra pathways of which two, the Ren and Chong channels, are particularly connected to women's reproductive health and with the ability to conceive. They can provide a focus for treatment of some causes of infertility.

By inserting needles at particular points along the meridians, in order to stimulate the flow of energy and have an impact on the different systems or parts of the body they serve, acupuncture seeks to correct any imbalances. In understanding this it is possible to see how acupuncture can have quite a dramatic effect on a variety of problems.

One example featured in a report published in the *Nursing Times* in 1988 (Robinson, Infertility and Subfertility) showed that acupuncture had been useful in the treatment of pelvic inflammatory disease. And a report published in *Gynaecological Endocrinology* in 1992 suggested that auricular acupuncture (acupuncture applied to specific points of the ear) seemed to offer a valuable alternative therapy for female infertility due to hormone disorders.

'I'm afraid I was rather a sceptic when it came to alternative medicine. But when we discovered that I didn't always ovulate, and that Peter's sperm count was a bit on the low side, the only option seemed to be drugs to give my hormones a bit of an oomph. I didn't fancy this, so thought I would give acupuncture a go before trying drugs. For me, the effect was almost immediate although I don't think this is the same for everyone. And I felt much more well, generally, which is partly why I was so keen to continue. I went weekly for about two months, by which time I was pregnant. Apart from my periods arriving on the dot of 28 days while I was having treatment, I actually don't know whether or not it was the acupuncture that helped. But we had been trying, albeit haphazardly, for over three years before we saw our doctor, let alone the acupuncturist.'

Mary, aged 29

You are likely to need a series of visits for acupuncture, and the cost of this can range from £40 to £75 per time. The first consultation will be the longest, because of the need to take a full history, while subsequent visits are likely to be shorter. Some acupuncturists also prescribe Chinese herbal medicines to complement the acupuncture, which may incur an additional cost, or even some complementary homeopathic remedy. This will depend largely on the practitioner's range of skills and expertise. However, acupuncture is less likely to be covered by private health insurance, although this is worth checking if you already have cover.

Many doctors and nurses now have qualifications in acupuncture, so you may find this service available to you through your local health practice. Qualified acupuncturists are registered with their official body. One last point to mention is that all needles used are disposable, so there is no risk of cross infection.

SHIATSU

Shiatsu, or acupressure, works on similar principles to acupuncture but involves the use of finger-tip pressure rather than needles. For this reason many people find it preferable. Its application and usage are relevant in treating some problems associated with infertility and subfertility and because, in company with other complementary therapies, it supports both the physical and the psychological, is beneficial in promoting positive health.

Qualified shiatsu practitioners are registered with the Shiatsu Society through which you should be able to find someone practising locally. Finding someone with skill and expertise is important because like other complementary therapies, shiatsu can be a powerful tool and has to be carefully used, particularly where there is a history of repeated miscarriage, for example. Most shiatsu practitioners will avoid treating a woman during the first three months of her pregnancy.

Costs of treatment vary, but usually average at between £40 to £75 per visit. You can expect to feel the benefit of treatment immediately if you suffer some sort of acute problem, although the long-term benefits are usually dependent on some sort of sustained treatment over time.

AROMATHERAPY

The therapeutic use of essential oils, and the utilisation of their medicinal qualities, is fast gaining in popularity. What was previously dismissed as a beauty therapy is being evaluated, especially as numerous research studies show that it is more than the massage that is effective: properties of the essential oils have definite therapeutic effects. Although the oils can be applied in a variety of ways, seldom neat, the most common practice is to add them to a carrier oil and apply to the skin in conjunction with the benefits of body massage.

There is no doubt that stimulating the sense of smell has in turn an effect on an area of the brain known as the limbic system. This is connected to our emotional behaviour, and the link between strong emotions and the release of various body chemicals is well established. For example, fear can create a rush of adrenalin, making the pulse race. The effect of aromatherapy on the limbic system can stimulate the release of hormones in the body. This can be used, by a skilled aromatherapist, to beneficial effect in fertility problems.

A qualified aromatherapist will select different essential oils that have a particular therapeutic effect, specific to an individual's needs. Either one or several will be blended in a carrier oil prior to application. For example, geranium is thought to help regulate hormones, and could be combined with melissa and rose oils, also known to be relevant to treating problems with conception. While with men, jasmine is thought to have a beneficial effect on the production of sperm.

It may be that you have sought the help of an aromatherapist for a specific diagnosed problem linked to an apparent inability to conceive, or because you want to utilise its effectiveness in helping you deal with stress, or anxiety related to an apparent inability to conceive, or just because you feel it may be a useful adjunct to dealing with infertility treatment. The hands-on effect of massage can be therapeutic in itself, but it is the specific therapeutic effects of the essential oils, carefully selected by a skilled practitioner that are of individual and particular benefit.

You can expect an aromatherapy session to last for between forty-five minutes to an hour and a half, and payment will in part depend on the length of the session. Costs vary from between £20 to £45, and although a one-off aromatherapy massage can be beneficial, for long-standing problems you would need to have a course of treatment, possibly once a week for four weeks and then fortnightly, and then once a month to keep the benefit going. So there is considerable investment to be made, and the choice is a personal one. The cost of treatment does not always include the cost of the essential oils used, so this needs to be borne in mind too.

Finding a qualified and aromatherapist can be done through the Aromatherapy Organizations Council. Treatment given by an aromatherapist can be extended at home, following their advice, through the use of essential oils in vapourisers or in the bath, or in using appropriate oils in a carrier and giving and receiving a massage from your partner.

REFLEXOLOGY

Based on the principle that different focal areas of the hands and feet correspond to different organs or systems of the body, then by massage and manipulation of these areas it is possible to treat disorders and disease. It is also possible to diagnose areas of weakness and detect problem areas that have arisen in the past or may cause a problem in the future.

The use of reflexology for problems with conception is, as with acupuncture, quite relevant because it is possible to indirectly stimulate specific organs.

'I had a diagnosed problem with my level of progesterone, following two early miscarriages, it was very low and so I had treatment with Clomid and IVF, but no further pregnancy had resulted. I originally went to see a reflexologist in order to try and help my body cope naturally and, after the disappointment of medical treatment, didn't hold out much hope. The reflexologist worked on the pituitary area, to balance my hormones and also directly on the area linked to my womb and ovaries. I was also given a Bach flower remedy, Crab Apple, to help relieve my negative thoughts. My first

reflexology session helped enormously in relieving my tension and anxiety about everything so I continued to see her and, without medical treatment – we were waiting for another IVF attempt – I conceived three months later.'

Kelly, aged 31

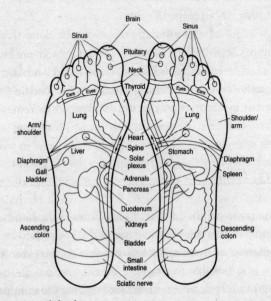

Reflexology points of the feet

You can expect a first consultation to last for over an hour, because of the need to take a comprehensive case history before treatment starts. Subsequent treatments should last about an hour, and the cost per session can range from £40 to £75. Some people have found initial treatments quite painful, as work on breaking down crystalline deposits at specific reflex points begins. This also depends in part on how sensitive your feet are and for some, reflexology is hopeless because they do not like having their feet handled at all.

You may want to utilise reflexology to improve your general reproductive health prior to conception, or because you know of a particular problem that could benefit from help or you have a diagnosis of unexplained infertility. In any event, you will need the skills of a qualified practitioner, who you can contact via the Association of Reflexologists.

HERBAL MEDICINE

The use of medicinal herbs is a healing art which pre-dates contemporary medicine. Many drugs today are based on plant extracts where the active components are utilised to treat specific symptoms, whereas herbal medicine uses the whole plant in its remedies. Like other alternative therapies, herbalism works by promoting the body's own healing systems, although they have specific ways in which they are used and, as a consequence, classified. Classification of a herbal remedy is described in terms of its effect; for example, anti-spasmodic, sedative, tonic, demulcent, stimulant, to name a few. Herbal remedies can be administered in a variety of ways, through infusions, decoctions, compresses, tinctures or douches.

A herbal remedy may involve one or several herbs taken together, depending on the prescriptive advice of the medical herbalist. For example, herbs to regulate the menstrual cycle may be combined with those to improve circulation to the organs of the reproductive system. Or herbs to reduce post-infection inflammation could be combined with those to stimulate the ovaries. There are also herbs recommended for the stimulation of sperm production.

Costs of treatment vary, and may or may not include the cost of any herbal medicine or tincture. A herbalist may charge more for a first session, as this is likely to be longer and needs a comprehensive personal history taken. Costs can range from £40 to £75, but any treatment on the NHS is unlikely.

Herbals are potentially toxic if incorrectly administered, and consulting a medical herbalist who is properly trained and qualified is important. The holistic approach of medical herbalism means that all advice and prescriptions are tailored to your individual needs. The

National Institute of Medical Herbalists can provide you with a list of members if you cannot find one listed locally.

TRADITIONAL CHINESE MEDICINE

Practitioners make a diagnosis based on Chinese principles of health, which are quite different from Western medicine. As with acupuncture, there is the same emphasis on the Qi (life force), and the balance between Yin and Yang. In addition, traditional Chinese medicine uses a diagnostic system based on eight principles by which disorders and diseases can be described. And the overall approach is holistic; the body is considered in the light of an individual's symptoms, age, temperament and lifestyle. Treatment might consist of acupuncture, massage, dietary advice and the use of herbal medicines.

Reports published over the last few years show that a number of studies of men being treated by traditional Chinese herbal medicine have improved their sperm count and motility. While orthodox medicine can offer little to improve the quality and quantity of a man's sperm, some alternative therapies and this one in particular can be helpful.

Costs vary, especially with the cost of pills or infusions, but range between £40 and £75. You can expect the first consultation to take a good hour, and concentrate very much on compiling a thorough medical and personal history, although the questions asked will reflect the principles of Chinese rather than Westernised medicine. You may find that your acupuncturist also practises Chinese herbal medicine, too, or vice versa. And some doctors trained in China will have embraced both the orthodox and the traditional disciplines of medicine, and may practise in both areas.

Herbal medicine can be extremely potent, and toxic, and should only be prescribed by a qualified and registered practitioner in traditional Chinese medicine. You can consult the Register of Chinese Herbal Medicine, and may find a registered practitioner within your vicinity, although they are less prolific than other alternative health practitioners.

NATUROPATHY

Naturopathic practitioners use a variety of treatments to influence and enhance the body's own ability to heal itself. These treatments include dietary modifications, fasting, hydrotherapy, exercise and often the use of manipulative or soft tissue techniques like osteopathy. The basic principles of a healthy life – a balanced diet of nutritious food and pure water, plenty of fresh air and exercise, and adequate rest – create the starting blocks of good health. Although this seems quite simple, most of us live a life that contains a good degree of stress and imbalance which, for most of the time we can effectively 'get away with'.

When dealing with a particular set of physical or emotional circumstances, and this can include trying to conceive a baby, then it may be well worthwhile to try and improve not just the possibility of pregnancy but also that this should be a positive experience in terms of health and fitness.

A naturopath will devise a particular plan of treatment individual to each patient. This may include a number of blood and urine tests in order to define what might be necessary in terms of dietary changes, nutritional supplements and herbal medicines. Treatment is also designed to detoxify the body, and revitalise its ability to self-heal. Often patients who embark on a course of naturopathic treatment experience what is described as a 'healing crisis' after a few weeks of treatment, where the symptoms treated become much worse before getting better. This is an anticipated part of the process.

Costs for naturopathic treatment do not come cheap, partly because of the comprehensive and individual nature of treatment, and can vary between £40 and £75 per session. You can expect the first consultation to be both the longest and most expensive, and also bear in mind that the costs of any clinical tests and prescribed herbs or homeopathic remedies may be extra.

Practitioners have to undergo a four-year training, prior to registration with the General Council and Register of Naturopaths (see Useful Addresses). Always check that any practitioner you visit is registered and, if not sure, you can always contact the General Council direct to check.

MASSAGE

Massage can be extremely useful not just in itself, but also as an adjunct to other therapies, in both alleviating muscle tension and facilitating relaxation. That in itself is a useful method of reducing stress and anxiety levels. Massage can vary quite dramatically in both its execution and its impact. The massage offered at your local health and beauty parlour is only really as good as the beauty therapist. It may be enough, or may leave you feeling that a more holistic massage might be of greater benefit.

Massage ranges so considerably in its intensity, from the traditional Swedish massage techniques to the deep tissue massage designed to relieve knots in muscles, or that designed to stimulate oriental massage points. It is important to talk through the techniques used before you start, and be sure you understand the way in which a particular masseur works. The very deep massage, for example the Chinese *tuina*, can be quite painful to start with. It is designed to actually unblock energy channels, through a pushing and twisting motion into the muscles.

Whichever approach or technique your selected masseur uses, some aspects of massage remain the same. You can expect to spend over an hour on a session, although less time may be given to a personal or medical history as a masseur will expect to discover a lot about how things are physically from actually working on your body. You should be treated in a warm, private environment that enables you to feel relaxed before you start. Massage oil is usual, either with or without the addition of scented or essential oils. The carrier oil should be vegetable-based, and light enough to be easily absorbed. At the end of a massage you should feel both relaxed and reinvigorated, and take things easy for an hour afterwards. For most people, the immediate benefits of massage are quite tangible and these should last for some time. Over a period of time, with regular massages, the benefits should be accumulative.

There is no doubt that hands-on and touch-based therapies like massage are wonderfully therapeutic. The sensory stimulation can actually enhance the body's immune system, raise the level of endorphins produced by the brain which heighten mood and generally create a feeling of well-being, all of which is greatly beneficial.

'I was lucky to find a masseur, recommended by a friend, who used a variety of approaches, from cranial osteopathy, to deep tissue massage to reiki, which is a Japanese form of healing touch. This meant that she adapted her massage techniques to what my particular needs were. They was nothing specifically 'wrong' with me, apart from a long-standing minor back problem, but I certainly felt enormously better all over after a series of weekly sessions. She came to my home and it was the best of all possible treatments for me, £60 for well over an hour.'

Catherine, aged 34

Anyone can offer massage, as a beauty or health therapy, and the service is completely unregulated. This does mean that the onus is on you to check up on the training and credentials of the masseur you use. The British Massage Therapy Council, established in the UK in 1992, is setting up a register which should make finding a reputable practitioner easier. Also in the UK is the Massage Therapy Institute of Great Britain, which lists those practitioners whose training and expertise they recognise, who can help and advise you.

Costs vary depending on what is offered and where, and how long a session is. Expect to pay a little more if a masseur is prepared to come to your home to treat you. Charges can range from between £40 to £75, so check what you can expect to pay.

HEALING

Healing is poorly understood in its effectiveness, but very effective it can be. In the UK there are over 20,000 healers of various sorts, working in a variety of ways. The general principle is that healing energy is all around us and what a healer does is to channel it. Different descriptions for different types of healing exist, but the most common phrase used is spiritual healing, where the 'power' to focus healing energy is thought to come from a divine source. While some healing is done very much in a hands-on way, it is also possible for distance healing to be effective. And it does not matter whether or not you believe it will work for healing to be effective. While some healers believe it is a gift that they have, others believe that the healing potential is present in all of us and it just requires practice and tuning in order to utilise it to good effect.

The four main healing approaches are:

- spiritual healing, which usually involves the laying on of hands, or through distance healing;
- *reiki*, used to rebalance energy channels in a patient through the energy emitted by the healer's hands, although this can also be done from a distance;
- therapeutic touch, which is similar to spiritual healing although the healer works just above a patient's body, 'unruffling' the energy field surrounding the body to rebalance and energise it. Originating from the US, it is practised by many traditionally-trained nurses and is particularly useful for relaxation and self-healing;
- faith healing, usually operating through a church, or prayer groups and has a religious aspect.

The occasions when some form of healing might be beneficial to help conception are many. It may be that conception just is not happening, even though there is no diagnosed reason why not. Or it may be that you are recovering from some infertility treatment, for example a laparoscopy, and want to enhance your body's recovery. Chronic ailments like endometriosis may be another reason to consult a healer.

'I used to turn up for a session with Sue feeling, literally, all over the place. There was no point me trying to tell her how I was feeling, because she could 'read' my body better than I could myself. Through a combination of massage and reiki I would feel things beginning to flow more easily again as she worked on my body. I had first gone to see her following a torn ligament in my leg after a skiing holiday, which wasn't improving as fast as I'd liked, then I got into the habit of seeing her off and on when I felt I needed grounding. When we were having problems conceiving, it made sense for both of us to have some sessions with her – I am sure it helped.'

Catherine, aged 42

Many healers already work in a more traditional way, perhaps as a masseur, aromatherapist or osteopath, using one discipline to enhance the other. In any event, like any holistic approach, they will adapt their practice to suit their patient's needs.

Many healers don't charge for their work, believing that they have a duty to utilise their God-given gift. Otherwise, expect to pay a fee in the region of £40 to £60 for a first session, perhaps paying less for subsequent visits. Occasionally healing is available, following referral by your doctor, on the NHS and is worth asking about if you think it may be for you.

Contact the umbrella organisation, the Confederation of Healing Organisations for further information. Avoid anyone who promises to cure you, they are going against the CHO's code of professional conduct, and can be struck off. The National Federation of Spiritual Healers is the largest organisation in the UK, with over 7,000 members, and can be contacted for general advice and also for a contact near you.

8 Assisted conception

'The dawning realisation that, without help, we wouldn't be able to have a child, was difficult to take on board. Although I felt quite positive about our chances, my heart sank as I began to understand what it would all mean.'

Eileen, aged 38

For some couples the only solution to their problems in trying to conceive a baby may be assisted conception, in one form or another. Assisted conception describes a number of processes where, for a variety of reasons, conception cannot occur under 'normal' circumstances: through sexual intercourse. The reasons why assisted conception may be a possible solution for a couple will be entirely individual and specific to them. What is important is that a full and relevant diagnosis should be a precursor to decisions made about assisted conception, which is why it is usually a conclusion arrived at after considerable time and investigation. And, because of the physically, emotionally and often financially demanding requirements of these procedures, it is not a decision to be arrived at lightly.

Even when decisions about opting for assisted conception have been made, this is only the beginning of a long journey. Availability of treatment in the UK is mixed, and NHS options are limited. Some clinics, NHS or private have policies about not treating single women, or unmarried couples. For a couple already coping with the anxiety and sadness infertility may have invoked, these restrictions seem cruel indeed. Lack of resources for couples facing infertility is a big issue, and the organisation doing most to try and change things, and support individuals in the meantime, is the Infertility Network UK, and AC-CESS in Australia (see Useful Addresses).

Apart from the relatively straightforward artificial insemination, assisted conception is also something of a 'last resort', because of the reasons outlined above. It is often a treatment that has to be repeated on numerous occasions, with no successful outcome guaranteed. Success rates in general can seem low, although the average success rate for any one treatment is influenced in part by the specialist centre where it is carried out. If you are trying to evaluate the success of one clinic against another just by their statistics this can be quite difficult because so many different factors have to be taken into account. These factors include:

- the specific cause of infertility that gave rise to treatment;
- whether there is a problem in both partners;
- the length of time there has been an infertility problem;
- whether a couple have had any previous pregnancies, independent of outcome;
- the number of previous treatment cycles;
- whether a treatment cycle was stimulated or unstimulated.

However, figures from the Human Fertilisation and Embryology Authority (HFEA) for 2006 showed that the number of women having successful in vitro fertilisation (IVF) treatment topped 10,000 for the first time. There were 10,242 births resulting in 12,596 babies in 2006, an increase of 13.1% on the number of births in 2005.

Live birth rates (the percentage of live births per treatment cycles started) also rose – 23.1% of treatments resulted in a live birth in 2006, up 1.5% for on the previous year. In 1992, the first year the HFEA started collecting data, the live birth rate was just 13%. The number of patients and the number of treatments also increased. These 2006 figures showed that 34,855 women were treated at UK clinics – an increase of 6.8% on the previous year – and underwent 44,275 cycles of treatment.

Overall success rates increased in every age group. For women under 35 using their own freshly collected eggs, the live birth rate was 31% compared to 29.6% in 2005. For women over 44 using their own fresh eggs, the rate increased from 0.8% in 2005 to 4% in 2006. What did fall, however, were the rates of multiple births – the biggest health risk for mothers and babies after IVF – from 24% of all births in 2005, to 22.7% in 2006.

Donor insemination treatments were down 28%, with 4,225 treatments carried out in 2006 compared to 5,865 in 2005, although overall success rates for donor insemination were up slightly – 10.8% of treatments resulted in a live birth compared to 10.3% in 2005.

The best source of up-to-date information for all licensed clinics in the UK is the Human Fertilisation and Embryology Authority (HFEA) (see Useful Addresses), who provide free *Infertility: The HFEA Guide*, which is essential reading for anyone contemplating assisted conception. Certainly it is a mistake for any couple finding themselves at the beginning of a process of investigation to think that any problem they may have can be easily solved through assisted conception. It is often a long, arduous and disappointing process. That is the downside. But for more and more couples, assisted conception has made parenthood a reality, especially as techniques improve. Like so much else, information is key and finding out what is and is not possible for *you* is imperative, in order to work out what options might exist. Reading this book is perhaps part of this process, while other resources include your doctor, infertility specialist, specially trained counsellors, self-help groups like the Infertility Network, and the HFEA.

'If I had known then what I know now about what is required to conceive through IVF, I would have thought long and hard about embarking on the route to parenthood via assisted conception. It was worth it, in the end, but it was fraught with difficulties.'

Tina, aged 39

'It wasn't the actual treatment that was problematic, just the thought that we needed it in the first place. I didn't want anyone to know, at all, and that made it difficult with our families because we were on such a rollercoaster of emotions throughout the four attempts at IVF.'

Grace, aged 33

'I had always known that having children was going to be something of a problem, because I'd had appendicitis followed by peritonitis at seventeen, leaving both Fallopian tubes badly scarred. What was interesting as I became older, was seeing my chances improve as technology got better. As IVF was my only option, I just felt fortunate that over the preceding ten years, it had become more likely to work by the time I needed it. And I was lucky, I conceived twins at my second attempt, and they are now four and thriving.'

Anurada, aged 32

It cannot be stressed too strongly that the reasons for problems in conceiving, and the possible solutions, are completely individual to the woman or couple involved. Drawing conclusions from someone else's experience, or making comparisons with another, have little to recommend them overall. Trying to fully understand your own situation, what options may be available and how these may come together to create a solution for you, is completely individual. Arm yourself with all the information you can, ask questions if you do not understand, but make sure that you are aware of what is specific and pertinent to you. There is a great potential for assisted conception, but it also has its limitations. Understanding both sides of this particular coin can be helpful as you work towards what might be successful for you.

There are five main forms of assisted conception: artificial insemination (with either donor or partner's sperm); in-vitro fertilisation (IVF); gamete intra-fallopian transfer (GIFT); egg donation; and micro-assisted fertilisation (MAF). While some elements of these techniques exist in common, for example, egg extraction or embryo transfer, reasons why one technique is selected over another can be the result of several considerations, the most pertinent of which is the couple's own personal situation.

ARTIFICIAL INSEMINATION

Artificial insemination by donor sperm is usually done because the male partner's sperm is either non-existent, or not of sufficiently good quality for conception to occur. Advances in some reproductive technologies have made it more possible for men whose sperm is of poor quality to still father a child, through techniques like IVF (see pages 127–31) or sub-zonal insemination (SUZI) (see page 133) and intra-cytoplasmic sperm injection (ICSI) (see page 133) which are forms of micro-assisted fertilisation (MAF).

In addition, women who want to have a child on their own, or in partnership with another women, might want to select this process in order to achieve pregnancy. Or donor insemination is sometimes used when there is a genetically inherited problem that a couple do not wish to pass on to their unborn child.

In some instances donor insemination is the only option available for couples where the man has been paralysed from the waist down and, in 85% of cases, the man can no longer ejaculate. Some progress with new techniques of electro-ejaculation, pioneered by the Royal National Orthopaedic Hospital, Stanmore and University College Hospital, London, means that DI will no longer be the only option in these cases as techniques develop and facilities improve.

Around ninety centres for donor insemination (DI) exist in the UK, although not all these provide treatment on the NHS. These centres have to be licensed by the Human Fertilisation and Embryology Authority (HFEA), and there are certain statutory obligations that have to be fulfilled. Issues of confidentiality are very strictly adhered to, and information that is recorded at the centre about donors or recipients cannot be disclosed except under legally-defined circumstances.

There is quite a comprehensive consultative process recommended, prior to DI treatment, which provides an opportunity to discuss a couple's, or individual's, personal and medical reasons for donor insemination. Counselling is sometimes recommended, in order to try and ensure that any residual grief is addressed, and that a couple fully understand the implications – emotional, social and legal – of what donor insemination means to them.

'It absolutely didn't matter to me that, biologically, someone else had given my son life. From the moment Jenny knew she was pregnant, I just felt happy and pleased to know that we had been given this chance to be parents. Not for one moment do I ever think my children are not 'mine'. We have just been so fortunate to create our own family, it was one of the reasons Jenny and I married, so it was important to each of us individually but also as part of our marriage.'

Gary, aged 29

'I found the whole business of donor insemination troubling. I can't quite put my finger on it, whether it is my own deep-seated feelings of inadequacy or because I felt that being pregnant was more important to my wife than were my feelings. It is very complex for me. Sometimes when I feel angry with my son, who is now eleven I can't tell whether this is 'normal' or because at some level I am angry with him for not being wholly my child, and what he represents in my life.'

Simon, aged 42

Donors are carefully selected and screened. Semen is tested and frozen and stored for six months until results are conclusive. This is obviously important to avoid any inadvertent transmission of disease, or HIV (human immuno-deficiency virus), for example. Physical characteristics of the donor are noted, in an effort to match donors in terms of hair and eye colouring, height, ethnic background, etc.

Any mother of a child by donor insemination is the legal mother, and her husband or partner is the legal father as long as he has consented to this treatment. There is no legal obligation to tell a child his true origins, although many parents are clearly informative about this, and opt to tell their child or children at an appropriate age. It is likely that the social father's name is entered on the birth certificate, although if he is not married to the baby's mother he has to go with her to the registrar to register the birth in order for his name to appear.

'I had always wanted children, but I wanted them to be brought up in a loving partnership. As a lesbian, I grew up wondering how possible this was going to be for me. My partner was happy for me to experience the pregnancy and birth, but wasn't keen on our knowing exactly who the father was. I felt quite divided about this because, at one level, I believe that it is every child's right to know their biological background, and yet at another I didn't want to have to "share" any child born to us with someone we knew. Friends of mine said it wouldn't matter in the long run, but I felt we had to try and work out what was best in the future for us and any child we might have, at this point of decision-making. Eventually, we opted for DI through a clinic and that worked very well. Now, two children and seven years later we are a close-knit and happy family. How they actually came about seems immaterial, and we have explained it to them in as simple and straightforward manner as we can, given their age. No doubt questions will come up again and again over the years to come, but the children seem very happy and accepting now.'

Sylvie, aged 39

Artificial insemination using the husband's, or partner's, sperm (AIH) is rarely useful where there is a low sperm count, although it is sometimes recommended. Regular sexual intercourse, combined with closer attention to the time of ovulation in a woman, is probably just as effective and may be less stressful for a couple's relationship.

Occasionally, where difficulties in achieving full sexual intercourse occur, then AIH may be suggested. And where there is some problem with the shape or position of the womb which might be hindering fertilisation and conception, this may also be an occasion when AIH is used.

The actual process of insemination is quite straightforward: a freshly collected sample of semen is collected and inserted high into the woman's vagina. For optimum results, the procedure is designed to coincide with when a woman is ovulating. If pregnancy occurs, it should follow a normal course with no increased risk of miscarriage or other problems, including congenital abnormalities.

Sometimes when a husband or partner's sperm count is considered poor, insemination of sperm directly into the uterus, via the cervix, is carried out. If this technique is used, sperm have to be collected and prepared in the laboratory before use. This procedure may sometimes be used where a woman has a problem with her cervix, or there is some evidence to suggest her cervical mucus is having an adverse effect on her partner's sperm.

While insemination is usually done under clinical conditions, self-insemination at home is perfectly possible. However, one of the drawbacks of this informal arrangement, where donor sperm has been supplied by someone known to the woman or couple, is that there is no health screening of the sperm or any legal protection for either party. More pertinently, perhaps, are the future implications for any child born this way. These issues have to be carefully weighed up by any prospective parent and informal donor.

IN-VITRO FERTILISATION

This technique is commonly referred to as 'test-tube' conception, where an egg from the woman is fertilised by the man's sperm before being replaced in the womb. It is a treatment originally devised to enable women with either blocked or damaged Fallopian tubes to conceive. In these cases, there is no possibility of the sperm and egg meeting, or a fertilised egg travelling to the womb for implantation. Today the procedure may also be suggested where a woman produces antibodies to her partner's sperm, preventing conception, where she has hormonal problems, or even for cases of apparently unexplained infertility.

It is, however, a complex and demanding procedure both emotionally and physically. In addition, the availability of IVF will depend largely on the area in which you live, or your ability to pay for private treatment. NHS waiting lists can be long, where couples could face a wait of up to three years. After the age of thirty-five it is also unusual for women to be offered NHS treatment.

Once the decision has been made, after extensive medical tests and consultation in most circumstances, selection for an IVF programme of treatment is only the first step. The IVF team working with a couple need to ensure that all aspects of the sequence of events leading up to possible conception are fully understood. This consultative process is very important, and may also involve the time and skills of a clinic counsellor who can help a couple cope with the emotional side of treatment. This is important not only because of the high hopes invested in IVF and the possible disappointments, but also because of the heavy demands IVF can make on a couple's relationship.

The first stage in an IVF cycle is to suppress the secretion of oestrogen, in order to dampen its effect on the ovaries, and this usually starts just after the beginning of a period. This suppressant is given daily, either via a nasal spray, or a sub-cutaneous (under the skin) injection, and can be self-administered at home. Ultrasound checks on the ovaries are made between two to three weeks later and if this first drug regime has worked, and the ovaries have been suppressed, then a second drug treatment begins. The primary purpose of this initial suppression of the ovaries is to make their response to the subsequent drug treatment more effective.

This second drug treatment is designed to stimulate not just one ovarian follicle, but several, in order to finally produce a number of eggs. Through blood tests and ultrasound monitoring, it is possible to judge when the developing follicles are sufficiently mature, before another drug is given to stimulate ovulation. This drug is given thirty-six hours before egg collection, at the point at which the ripe eggs are about to be released.

'I don't know how we got through those weeks of hormonal work-up for the egg collection. It threw me badly, and I was all over the place – moody, tearful, irritable and downright angry – describing the possible side-effects as feelings of moodiness was the understatement of the year in my case. Luckily the number of eggs collected meant that we ended up with five embryos, enough for two attempts. And we were lucky, it worked!'

Alexa, aged 32

Egg collection can be done either under general anaesthetic or sedation. Sedation is used more frequently, with access to the ovary via the vagina and Fallopian tube while using ultrasound. Each mature egg removed from the follicle is individually extracted using a gentle suction device. It is usual to remove as many eggs as are mature and available. These are then placed in a jelly-like fluid, the culture medium, in a glass dish and stored in an incubator.

Freshly-produced sperm from the woman's partner is then mixed with these eggs. It is likely that the semen sample from the man has been checked and treated to ensure a good number of moving, healthy sperm prior to this. It takes about eighteen hours for fertilisation to occur, and about twelve hours later the embryo starts to divide. Embryo transfer does not occur until two, if not three days in some clinics, after the eggs were collected and fertilised, by which time the embryos should have divided at least twice more. Doctors can examine the embryos microscopically and be sure that fertilisation has really occurred because, occasionally, eggs can divide without having been fertilised. Transferring these for implantation will be of no use at all.

Transfer of the embryos is done using an extremely fine piece of plastic tubing. Up to three fertilised eggs are sucked into the tube in their surrounding culture medium, and the tube is gently inserted into the womb, via the vagina and cervix, before being squirted out.

This whole procedure is completely painless, if a little uncomfortable.

It is quite usual to place more than one fertilised egg back, in an attempt to ensure a pregnancy occurs, but the HFEA's Code of Practice has stipulated that no more than three embryos should be replaced because of the health risks to the mother and her unborn babies. There is a much higher incidence of premature birth, complications in pregnancy and low birth weight with multiple births. Twins have an average birth weight of 2.5 kg, while for triplets the average birth weight is 1.8 kg, compared to 3.5 kg for single babies. Health problems in later life are more common in low birth weight babies, as is the incidence of disability and neonatal death. Because the HFEA was set up to act in the interests of the unborn child, as well as its parents, this is an important consideration.

Once the embryos have been transferred to the womb, there is no particular reason to recommend resting in bed, although many women do feel anxious about moving about. Implantation occurs independent of movement, and the chances of conception at this point are just about the same as for a woman conceiving under normal circumstances. What is different, of course, is the whole emphasis that IVF gives to conception. So much is vested in its success that it is hard not to worry about whether what you do or do not do will improve your chances. It is not much help to be told that there is not anything you can do that will make much difference at this stage, but that is the reality of the situation.

Of the three embryos that are returned to the womb, not all may implant. A woman's chance of conceiving ranges between none, one, two or three embryos developing into fetuses. The chances of a multiple pregnancy is increased on an IVF programme, to 20%, for obvious reasons. And if all three embryos implant, a woman may be offered a selective termination for one, or even two, of the fetuses. These are quite serious considerations, and very difficult decisions to make should they arise. It is very important, therefore, to be adequately advised of all aspects of an IVF programme and to fully consider and talk through the implications for you, individually, and as a couple, of any future decisions you may need to make.

Although no more than three embryos are ever replaced, others may be available and those suitable can be stored for possible future use. Cryopreservation, the storing at temperatures below freezing, involves the use of liquid nitrogen and temperatures of −196 degrees centigrade. This has been shown to preserve embryos without demonstrable deterioration.

Prior to any IVF treatment, which includes the use and storage of collected eggs, sperm and possible embryos, written consent has to be given by both parties involved. Any eggs, sperm or fertilised embryos can only be used in accordance with that written consent, whether for a couple's own use or for donation to another couple. If a pregnancy arises from the donation of a fertilised embryo, then the child born is legally of the receiving parents, not of the donating parents.

During the course of treatment, the clinic also has a legal obligation to collect personal information about those participating in treatment. While this information held by the clinic is completely confidential, it is a legal requirement because the HFEA has an obligation to tell someone over the age of eighteen, should they ask in the future, whether they were born as a result of IVF.

Clinics that store fertilised embryos have to be licensed to do so. They are allowed to store frozen embryos for up to five years, after which they are discarded. Keeping the embryos for this length of time allows for the possibility of a couple having another IVF baby at a later stage. Or, a fertilised embryo can be donated to another couple, although only with the written consent of the donating couple. Embryos can also be used for research, again only if written consent is given.

IN-VITRO MATURATION

In-Vitro Maturation, or IVM, is a form of IVF where immature eggs are removed from the woman's ovaries, and matured under laboratory conditions before being fertilised and implanted. Although the initial results from this treatment were less successful initially, success rates are improving. For women with polycystic ovary syndrome, for whom the drug stimulation prior to egg collection might induce a rare but potentially fatal condition called ovarian hyperstimulation syndrome (OHSS), IVM also offers hope for assisted conception. In addition to which, without all the drugs necessary to produce numerous mature eggs, the costs of treatment are reduced.

GAMETE INTRA-FALLOPIAN TRANSFER

GIFT, or ZIFT (zygote intra-fallopian transfer) is a similar procedure to IVF insofar as eggs are collected and mixed with sperm outside the body. Up to three eggs are combined with fresh semen, then this mixture, rather than a fertilised egg, is inserted in the top of the Fallopian tube, which is obviously only possible if there is no problem with the woman's tubes. GIFT is a more complex procedure than artificial insemination, but slightly less so than IVF and it is thought that in some cases the Fallopian tube is more conducive to fertilisation than a glass dish.

GIFT can be a useful option for couples where there is some problem with the man's sperm, perhaps the quality and quantity are low, or there has been some question mark over the compatibility between the sperm and egg. And for some patients who have what is referred to as 'unexplained infertility', GIFT can sometimes be a solution. Although, once again it is your specific circumstances that will influence whether or not this treatment is for you.

MICRO-ASSISTED FERTILISATION

There are some instances where however often you bring a couple's sperm and eggs into contact, fertilisation just does not occur. This is usually because of immature or poor quality sperm.

Two main techniques exist that could remedy this. The first involves the injecting of several individual sperm through the external layer of cells, or zona, of the egg and this is referred to as subzonal insemination or SUZI. The second technique involves the injection of one single sperm actually into the cytoplasm of the egg, and is referred to as intra-cytoplasmic sperm injection or ICSI.

As can be imagined, this technique is extremely skilled and only possible because of the power of modern microscopes and manufacture of micro-equipment. For example, the micro-needle used to inject the sperm into the egg during ICSI is estimated to be twelve times thinner than a single human hair, while the size of an egg is estimated as being around seven times smaller than a printed full stop. It is an extraordinary procedure.

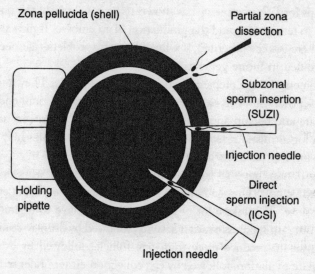

The SUZI and ICSI processes

Both these techniques form part of an IVF and embryo transfer programme, should they be the treatment of choice for a couple. As with all IVF treatment, the full medical work-up for egg collection remains the same, as is the procedure for embryo replacement in the womb. However, neither of these procedures are yet comprehensively available to all couples in the UK who may be suitable for treatment, partly because of the skill required but also because of its expense.

EGG DONATION

In the same way that some men are unable to produce sperm that can fertilise an egg, some women no longer – or never have been able to – produce eggs. Some women may have had to have medical treatment, perhaps for cancer treatment during childhood, involving the use of chemotherapy or radiotherapy. In these cases, their ovaries may have been damaged. In addition there are women whose egg production, perhaps for IVF treatment, has shown to be consistently too poor to result in fertilisation and the production of an embryo. It may also be that there is some inherited, sex-linked genetic problem that needs to be avoided in future generations.

Women who are prepared to donate eggs are scarce. They must be no older than thirty-five years, and HFEA guidelines recommend that they are and remain anonymous to the recipient. Volunteers usually do so for altruistic reasons, although some private clinics may offer some form of payment in terms of expenses.

Egg donors have to go through the same medical work-up as a woman on an IVF programme, in order to collect a number of eggs in due course. This asks a lot of a donor: she will have to tolerate the daily drugs to suppress ovarian activity, followed by drugs to stimulate the ovary to produce more than one follicle, followed by drugs to stimulate ovulation, followed by egg collection either under sedation or general anaesthetic. It is much to ask of someone, and those women who volunteer to donate their eggs are generous indeed.

'I decided that, because of the number of eggs that were collected for my own attempt at IVF, I would make a number available for donation. It was something my husband and I discussed and agreed, and talked through with *the clinic counsellor, when I started treatment. I think that deep down I felt that it was some sort of insurance policy, that I would be rewarded by this sharing of what I was able to produce so easily! Certainly we were able to conceive through IVF. Twice!'*

Gill, aged 30

Once a donor's eggs are collected, one of three things may happen. Three may be taken and mixed with the man's sperm before being replaced, prior to fertilisation, in his partner's Fallopian tube (GIFT with donor eggs); sperm and eggs may be mixed and, following confirmed fertilisation, up to three embryos may be inserted in the recipient's womb (IVF and embryo-transfer with donor eggs); or following the fertilisation of a donor's eggs, the resulting embryos may be frozen and stored to allow time to check for any problems including HIV status before transferring to the recipient's womb.

One very important feature of egg donation, and one that is similar to sperm donation, is the emotional aspect of this complex procedure. Careful thought and counselling is very necessary, both for the donor and recipient, and this is something that should be asked about if egg donation is mooted as a relevant option for you.

'At first I completely rejected the notion of egg donation. I felt so defeated as a woman, not being able to produce my own eggs, that opting for egg donation seemed to add insult to injury. It took me a long time to come round to the idea, and then it was only after a lot of talking it through with my partner. He was more concerned about me than my having a baby, and I think in some way because his priority was me, the idea became more acceptable. Then, of course, having decided to go ahead it all took forever to happen but I think it was better that way. I'm glad I waited until I felt really sure about what I wanted. It would have been awful to have been pregnant and still ambivalent about it all.'

Yvonne, aged 27

SURROGACY

Surrogacy is a limited option, and one that remains controversial. The situation in the UK is that while commercial surrogacy is illegal, as is the advertising for a surrogate or vice versa, actual surrogacy is not. It is, however, legal for a surrogate to receive some payment of expenses.

The reasons why a couple might consider using a surrogate mother are primarily where the woman has no internal reproductive organs to conceive or carry a child, or because her womb has been damaged, or surgically removed for some reason, although her ovaries remain intact.

Two main forms of surrogacy exist. The first is where a surrogate mother is artificially inseminated using the husband or partner's sperm; the second is where the surrogate mother carries the parents' genetic embryo, produced through IVF techniques, and is the 'host' mother for the duration of the pregnancy.

The former is the most common form of surrogacy currently occurring in the UK. All agreements are made on a private basis, and are not legally binding because the surrogate mother remains the 'legal' mother. This arrangement is wholly dependent on trust in order to succeed. Expenses for the mother, including those to cover the time of carrying the baby in the womb, can be paid legally.

Where a surrogate mother carries a couple's IVF-produced embryo, things become more complicated because they involve medical help and treatment. This treatment is unlikely to be available on the NHS, so the issue of cost is also involved. And, as before, however carefully thought out and drawn up the transaction is, it is not legally binding, and the surrogate mother remains entitled to keep the baby if she chooses to do so.

There are also other potential risks. As with any pregnancy, there is always the unknown factor of babies being born with previously unknown congenital or birth defects and being rejected by all its parents, or of the surrogate mother suffering in some way as a result of the pregnancy. COTS, the voluntary organisation involved in advising and supporting both infertile couples and surrogates (see Useful Addresses), reckon on there being around a 2% failure rate of the system as it currently stands. (This is not the same as the rate of conception which is linked to statistics for artificial insemination and IVF in general).

Surrogacy remains a particularly complex area for all concerned and, while there are couples for whom this has been an ideal and workable solution, it is not for everyone and requires extremely careful thought, advice and consideration.

COUNSELLING

Reproductive technologies and assisted conception techniques improve and become more comprehensively available as time goes on. However, they must be seen for what they are: an opportunity to assist in conception. They are not a panacea for all conception problems and each individual situation has to be carefully assessed.

While many, many couples who have an initial infertility problem go on to successfully have children, there will be some couples who never manage to conceive a longed-for child. It is a particularly hard sort of grief because, caught up with all the inability to fulfil dreams centred around what we consider to be family life, is the grief for someone who never actually existed, except within those all-important dreams – a child who was never actually conceived or born, and all the hopes and plans linked to that which cannot be fulfilled.

At any stage along the way with infertility investigations and treatments, each couple has to carry the burden of potential failure, until a child is conceived. This can place an enormous strain on an individual and also on a couple's relationship. This strain can become apparent at any stage along the way, and different things will trigger different responses in each partner. It is a situation that often requires the external help of a skilled and trained counsellor, who has experience of helping many couples in the same situation. If this service is offered to you, take it up even if you do not feel it to be immediately useful, as what you discuss may be beneficial further down the line; use it to explore some of the issues that will inevitably arise.

Any clinic that provides IVF, or treatment that involves donated sperm, eggs or embryos, must offer counselling. This is a legal requirement stipulated by the HFEA before a clinic's licence is granted. If your investigations or treatment are either not yet at this stage, or fall outside a specialist clinic's remit, you may not be offered any sort of emotional support. Ask your doctor about this, because there are other options. A GP practice or health centre may have access to a counselling service or may provide it themselves.

In any event, if you have reason to feel that you need help in coping with the impact of both infertility and its treatment, ask for it. Recognition of the difficulties couples face has grown over the years, and much more support is now available. Because of the taboo nature of infertility, it can be an extremely isolating experience, but there are people out there who do truly understand, not least because they have been through the experience themselves and now lend their support to others through infertility self-help groups like the Infertility Network (see Useful Addresses). It can help ease the feeling of isolation to talk to someone.

'As a couple we appeared to be coping fairly well, but it was an undercurrent of anxiety that was always there. Would we, wouldn't we, ever become parents? Could we, couldn't we, ever cope with it? These refrains were constant companions in my head for months. Sometimes I thought I would go mad if I couldn't get away from thinking about it all. It was wonderful to wake up every morning with a head empty of questions, appointments, calendar dates, but awful to feel the realisation begin to surface. Part of the joy of actually having a baby was not having to think about all this any more. If I hadn't seen a counsellor during this time, I'm not sure I could have held it together.'

Rhian, aged 37

*'At the time the excitement of actually trying to have a baby kept me going.
We both felt very positive about it all. Obviously when things didn't go our
way initially it was hard, but I never felt that it took over our lives.'*

Paula, aged 29

Alternatively, contact the Infertility Network, who provide a unique
telephone counselling service; or another body concerned with
infertility and problems in conception, the British Infertility Counselling Association, (see Useful Addresses).

9 Miscarriage

'I couldn't believe it when I miscarried at eleven weeks. My first pregnancy had been completely straightforward, no complications at all. It never occurred to me that something like this could happen and it was a tremendous shock. It completely undermined my confidence in my body's ability to carry a baby. Even though I'm now pregnant again, even at six months I still feel unsure in a way I didn't the first time around.'

Ellie, aged 28

'When I started to bleed at just gone ten weeks, I was concerned but not unduly. My pregnancy book said something about the possibility of a small bleed at around twelve weeks. But it didn't stop, so I went to the doctor's who sent me straight to the hospital for a scan. It was then that it became apparent things weren't quite right: there was in reality no baby, just what they call a blighted ovum. I miscarried completely within twenty-four hours. But it helped to know that I hadn't 'lost' an actual baby.'

Ginny, aged 32

For many women trying to have a baby, miscarriage or the threat of miscarriage can generate feelings of enormous grief and anxiety, whether or not a pregnancy has been straightforward or difficult to achieve. It can also be a very personal, and hidden grief, because very often no one, not even the closest of family or friends can fully understand about the hopes and dreams that were an integral part of early pregnancy. If miscarriage should follow assisted conception, with all the history of investigations and treatment this entails, then the emotional investment may somehow seem even greater.

The subject of miscarriage has been given a chapter of its own partly because of the significance of early pregnancy loss, but also because it can be an actual cause of infertility or, more accurately, because fertilisation and conception does occur, a cause of sub-fertility. In addition, for women who have difficulties conceiving in the first place, perhaps because of hormonal imbalances, these reasons may also contribute to an increased risk of miscarriage.

What also has to be stressed is that miscarriage is almost never a result of anything a woman has or has not done. While quite natural feelings of grief occur – sadness, questioning, self-blame, guilt, anger, depression – sometimes help is need to clarify and structure these, and counselling can be helpful when miscarriage occurs repeatedly, or even late in the pregnancy. Miscarriage is inevitably an emotional burden for a woman, but it can be equally so for her partner. What support a couple can give each other through this is dependent on the nature of their relationship, but for many couples it creates an additional strain that they are not always able to cope with. Being aware of this, and seeking external help if necessary, can help to strengthen existing communication. The support, advice and information offered by the Miscarriage Association (see Useful Addresses) can be invaluable.

Miscarriage can occur any time after a missed period to up to twenty-four weeks of pregnancy, after which it is referred to as stillbirth. Miscarriage is the most common complication of pregnancy: around 15% of all pregnancies end in miscarriage, and 25% of women who experience pregnancy will also experience at least one miscarriage.

Then there are the more positive statistics: if you have had just one miscarriage then the chances of the next pregnancy going to term are 80%; if you have had repeated miscarriages, and only 1% of women fall into this group, then you still have a 60% chance of your next pregnancy going to term.

Miscarriage is referred to, medically, as spontaneous abortion and can occur at any time during the first few months of pregnancy. For many women the actual causes remain unknown, and this can be particularly difficult to come to terms with. If it occurs up to three times consecutively, then it is referred to as habitual miscarriage, and referral for expert gynaecological advice is necessary. Even then it is not always possible to identify a specific cause, but support, advice and reassurance can be very helpful, and the majority of women do go on to have a baby successfully without medical intervention.

The medical use of the word 'abortion', even if it is preceded by the words 'spontaneous' or 'inevitable' can sound awfully harsh when the loss of a much-longed for baby is referred to in this way. In part, this is because our associations with the word abortion suggest a deliberate attempt to end a pregnancy, and when it is applied to the sadness of a miscarriage – whether early miscarriage before sixteen weeks, or a late miscarriage between sixteen and twenty-four weeks – it somehow makes the situation worse. Most doctors and nurses are more aware that the language they use can have this effect, even if they lapse into medical speak amongst themselves or write 'spontaneous abortion' on the medical notes.

SYMPTOMS OF MISCARRIAGE

Every woman who has a miscarriage will experience symptoms specific to her, although there are general signs common to all. One of the first of these will be vaginal bleeding. This may be a small amount of spotting or fresh blood, or a darker discharge if blood has been retained in the vagina for some time. Bleeding in itself not a sign of inevitable miscarriage: many women appear to lose quite large quantities of blood at some point in their pregnancy, with no apparent ill-effect to the baby.

It is worth remembering that some women experience spotting at the time an embryo implants in the lining of the womb, and this is called an implantation bleed which can occur during the first few weeks following conception, and can be confused with the beginning of a threatened miscarriage. In addition, some women may experience spotting again at around twelve weeks of pregnancy. This sometimes occurs when there is a small hormonal blip in the production of the pregnancy hormone progesterone which serves to keep the womb lining capable of nurturing a pregnancy. Initially produced by the ovaries, at around twelve weeks the maturing placenta takes over the production of progesterone, but the trigger for this is the slight falling-off of ovarian production. Any spotting around this time may be related to this.

If you do begin to bleed during early pregnancy, phone your GP for advice or, if you have been having any sort of infertility investigations or treatment, your specialist doctor. Having described your symptoms, you will probably be advised to rest in bed and see whether things settle down, which they very often do. Even women who have had quite substantial bleeds during early pregnancy can go on to success-fully carry their baby to term.

Another reason for checking with your GP about any bleeding in early pregnancy is dependent on the rhesus status of a mother's blood group.

While around 90% of the population are rhesus positive, if a mother has a rhesus negative blood group she will need an injection of something called anti-D within seventy-two hours of a miscarriage to prevent the formation of antibodies that could make a subsequent pregnancy difficult. For example, if you are blood group A rhesus negative, and your partner is blood group O rhesus positive, then the chances are that the fetus is a rhesus positive blood group too. This does not matter to either mother or baby while the pregnancy remains intact but, should there be any bleeding as with a miscarriage, by exposing the mother's blood supply to the fetus', the mother then develops antibodies to rhesus positive blood which will remain in her system forever, causing her no harm. Then, during a subsequent pregnancy, these existing antibodies will be hostile to the developing fetus' blood supply. It is a manageable situation, but one that is best and simply avoided by giving rhesus negative mothers an injection which prevents them creating the antibodies in the first place, following any childbirth, miscarriage or therapeutic abortion where an exchange of maternal and fetal blood can occur.

Bleeding when pregnancy is quite advanced, from around twenty weeks, may mean that there is a problem with the placenta. Some placentas are naturally low-lying in the womb. That is, they are attached to the lower portion of the womb rather than further up. In fact, during early pregnancy an ultrasound scan may have indicated this but it is not a problem because the position of the placenta 'moves up' the womb later on. It does not actually move, but the expansion of the womb occurs in such a way that the area below the placenta expands so the gap between it and the exit to the womb becomes greater. In a small proportion of women, around 3%, the placenta remains low-lying and as the womb expands during the normal course of pregnancy the lower edge of the placenta pulls away slightly which can give rise to some bleeding. While this needs to be reported, and monitored, it is not the same as a threatened miscarriage. What must also be borne in mind is that any bleeding is from the mother, and not from the baby.

Very often with a threatened miscarriage, particularly at a later stage of pregnancy, your doctor will request an ultrasound scan. This will give a good indication of how things are with the fetus. A fetal heartbeat can be picked up after about six weeks and, if this is the case, evidence suggests that around 90% of threatened miscarriages with a fetal heartbeat will not progress to inevitable miscarriage. If there is no apparent fetal heartbeat at the time of the first scan, a second scan a week later is usually suggested especially if the pregnancy is at a very early stage. If subsequent scans show no heartbeat, it is probably the death of the fetus that has caused the threatened miscarriage, which will then become inevitable.

'My heart was in my mouth when we went for our scan, to see whether the baby was all right. I hadn't bled very much, and they said it was a routine check because everything seemed to be OK, but I didn't believe it until I saw

my baby on the scan, and that strong heartbeat. It sort of gave me the confidence to believe we would make it.'

Simone, aged 34

The absence of a fetal heartbeat may also indicate that there was no pregnancy in the first place: and you may hear reference made to either a 'blighted ovum' or an 'anembryonic pregnancy'. Here, the placenta and amniotic sac have developed around an ovum that has failed to fertilise and develop normally. The pregnancy hormones are produced by the placenta, which is why the pregnancy appears to be progressing normally until this time.

The second likely symptom of miscarriage, which also suggests that it may become inevitable rather than just threatened, is abdominal pain coupled with continuing bleeding. Abdominal pain that is cramp-like, and feels similar to period pains, indicates that there is some dilatation of the cervix which suggests that miscarriage is inevitable and will complete its process over the next few days. Any symptoms of pregnancy, for example nausea and breast tenderness, may dramatically subside but this will depend on your own pregnancy symptoms and how far advanced the pregnancy was.

How pregnant you actually are will influence what you experience in terms of losing your baby. Very early miscarriage is relatively straightforward in physical terms: there will be some bleeding, possibly with large clots, and abdominal discomfort which should resolve itself within a few days. Some bleeding may continue for up to two weeks, but you will only need to contact your doctor again about this if it continues for longer, if the discharge becomes smelly and offensive, or if you become feverish. This may indicate an infection that needs treatment. An infection may mean that some of the pregnancy membranes have remained in the womb and need removing surgically with a D&C (dilatation and curettage), or as it is sometimes referred to, a 'scrape'. The other medical term you may hear used is evacuation of retained products of conception, an ERPC.

A later miscarriage will mean that, coupled with the above symptoms of bleeding and abdominal pain, you may actually be aware of delivering the gestational sac. This is the bag made of the amniotic membranes which contains the fetus. Whether or not this contains something recognisable as your baby depends on how advanced pregnancy was, or whether the fetus has been dead for some time, but what is self-evident is that this can only be enormously distressing psychologically as well as physically.

'Even though my miscarriage was relatively early, at sixteen weeks, I was unprepared for how painful it was. The abdominal contractions were very strong, producing terrible cramps. I had no choice but to take some painkillers and go to bed with a hot water bottle. Fortunately my doctor visited a couple of times and was very sympathetic, and I was able to be at home with my husband throughout.'

Stella, aged 30

A threatened miscarriage at a late stage may mean that you have been admitted to hospital for rest and care and, if miscarriage becomes inevitable, this is where it will occur. This may mean that you have the benefit of expert care and the opportunity for additional support and advice. It may also mean the reverse, particularly if you are on a gynaecological ward with a mixture of women with a variety of medical reasons for being there, including therapeutic abortion. Equally, if your pregnancy was well advanced you may have been actually on an obstetric ward, or an antenatal ward. Both of these circumstances can aggravate distress, so being at home may well be preferable, and a more secure place to grieve.

Following a miscarriage, you can expect to bleed for up to two weeks afterwards. This bleeding should diminish quite rapidly, but is more like a postnatal bleed, after the birth of a baby, than a period. It is probably better to use sanitary towels rather than tampons, to reduce any possibility of infection. And some would recommend showering rather than taking a bath initially, although there is unlikely to be any real risk of infection from bathing, especially in your own home. If the bleeding continues for longer than two weeks, or suddenly becomes more profuse after subsiding, or shows an increase in fresh blood, contact your doctor. Occasionally, not all the pregnancy comes away completely, running a small risk of infection and haemorrhage.

REASONS FOR MISCARRIAGE

While it is very often not possible to explain why a one-off miscarriage, or even why habitual miscarriage occurs, there are some reasons that are known about and for which treatment might be available. It is a natural need to try and find a reason for events like miscarriage, primarily in order to take steps to avoid a recurrence, but it is not always possible and that can make coming to terms with miscarriage very difficult. However, even when a possible cause is identified a subsequent pregnancy can proceed quite normally without treatment. It seems to be within the nature of conception that however much is known or understood, there remains an X factor that appears to either hinder all attempts to produce a healthy baby or conversely, contributes to something that can only be described as the miracle of life – when a baby is born against all seeming odds.

Chromosomal problems

A one-off miscarriage could be the result of a completely random problem that occurs during the early stages of cell division following fertilisation of the egg by the sperm. Half of all chromosomal information an embryo receives is from its mother, half from its father. If there is some hiccup in the early stages of cell division, an abnormal embryo results that is incapable of developing further and the pregnancy miscarries. Whether or not this happens is, as was said before, completely random which is why a first miscarriage for these reasons, although you may never be aware of its actual cause, is likely to be followed by a successful pregnancy.

One of the problems with this sort of miscarriage is that while there is no fetus developing normally, the placenta is continuing to develop as it should, and is also continuing to produce all the hormones that make a woman continue to feel pregnant. Not only that, but any pregnancy test will continue to test positive even though it is clear to the ultrasound technician that there is no developing fetus. It can be quite difficult to believe, and accept, that there is going to be no baby while still feeling so pregnant. Eventually miscarriage occurs between the eighth and eleventh week of pregnancy.

Very occasionally one partner may be the carrier for some sort of chromosomal abnormality which only becomes apparent when trying to conceive, and this may be the cause of recurrent miscarriages. This might affect between 3% and 5% of the 1% who repeatedly miscarry. So it is obviously only a very small number of couples who are affected by this. If it is possible to determine the nature and extent of any chromosomal abnormality, genetic counselling will enable a couple to understand the situation and what possible solutions there might be. These solutions may include IVF, in order to identify abnormal embryos before transferring back normal ones; or donor insemination (DI) if the problem lies with the man, for example.

Hormonal problems

Hormonal problems may have already been identified in a woman, perhaps because they have contributed to problems in conception that required treatment. The most significant of these is likely to be an over-secretion by the pituitary gland of luteinising hormone (LH). This is the hormone responsible for ovulation and too much of it is a feature of polycystic ovaries, where too many follicles try to ovulate immature eggs. If this has not been a cause of infertility problems it might arise now because the immature egg that is released, when fertilised, is unable to develop normally and miscarriage occurs.

Around 60% of women who repeatedly miscarry are found to have this problem. Diagnosis can be made from blood tests, in conjunction with ultrasound which can show whether the ovaries are polycystic. It may then be possible to treat hormonally, making the ovulation of an immature egg less likely.

Other hormonal imbalances which may cause repeated miscarriage may have already caused a history of endometriosis or sub-fertility. And the two hormones that are necessary for a pregnancy to continue once fertilisation and implantation have occurred, human chorionic gonadotrophin (hCG) and progesterone, may also be low in women who miscarry. Where these situations exist, a course of hormone injections given regularly over four weeks until the twelfth week of pregnancy may be the solution.

'Although I managed to conceive successfully, after a number of miscarriages my hormonal levels were checked. My levels of luteinising hormone (LH) were too low after ovulation to ensure that the corpus luteum developed adequately to produce enough progesterone to keep things going, until the placenta was mature enough to kick in . . . This didn't mean much to me except that I was then given hormone injections during the first few weeks, and they worked. It was such a relief to find out what the problem was, and then to find out that there was something that could be done!'

Mandy, aged 29

Auto-immune causes of miscarriage

In a small proportion of the 1% of women who suffer habitual miscarriage, around 15%, there may be a problem connected with the production of antibodies that make the blood clot more readily. When this occurs, clots can arise in the blood supply of the placenta reducing its ability to continue to nurture the fetus. If the damage caused by the blood clots is extreme, the fetus dies and the pregnancy miscarries. Because the effect of this blood disorder can take some time to reduce the efficiency of the placenta, it can be one of the reasons for late miscarriage, which is particularly distressing because the pregnancy is so far advanced and the miscarried baby so well-developed. Treatment for this cause of miscarriage is improving as research continues, and there is some evidence to show that regular low doses of aspirin, given under medical supervision, is effective.

Hughes Syndrome

Hughes Syndrome, also known as 'sticky blood' or 'Antiphospholipid Syndrome', is an autoimmune disease, which can cause abnormal blood clotting in any blood vessel, either arteries or veins. It also accounts for as many as 20% of recurrent miscarriages, thought to result from disruption of blood flow through the small blood vessels of the placenta. Although the exact sequence of events isn't yet clear (and may vary in each individual woman, and in individual pregnancies), this disruption of blood supply via the placenta means that the baby received inadequate nutrition and oxygen, and fails to thrive. Miscarriages that occur late in pregnancy are very strongly linked to Hughes Syndrome. The syndrome has also been linked to pre-eclampsia, placental abruption and intra-uterine growth restriction. For further information, contact the Hughes Syndrome Foundation (Useful Addresses).

Infections

A number of infections can cause miscarriage, among them German measles (rubella) which is one of the reasons why an immunisation programme exists for girls and why your rubella status is checked by one of the routine antenatal blood tests. Other infections which may increase the risk of miscarriage include toxoplasmosis and listeriosis. Although these infections are rare, advice is given in early pregnancy about avoiding known risks for these.

Vaginal infections can also be implicated in miscarriage, although not those which can be associated as a relatively normal common problem of pregnancy, for example, thrush. Any vaginal infection should be mentioned to your doctor in case it may cause a problem to the pregnancy, and treatment can be advised for both a woman and her partner in order to avoid the chance of re-infection.

One infection that is difficult to pick up, because it rarely produces symptoms that a woman can identify, is chlamydia. There is evidence to suggest that a chlamydia infection can be the cause of some infertility problems, ectopic pregnancy, miscarriage and premature labour. Although its effect can be profound, it is still relatively rare (it was only found in 7% of antenatal patients in one 1984 study [Wood et al]), and is tested for routinely. However, if a woman experiences repeated miscarriage, for no apparent reason, this may be something that she is tested for, and treatment is effective. While it is something that can be sexually transmitted, it can also be contracted from some farm animals, notably sheep. Unlikely though this is for most of us, for those who work with animals, avoiding this possible risk while pregnant is important.

In the UK, because chlamydia is currently the most commonly diagnosed sexually transmitted infection (STI) affecting both men and women, the National Chlamydia Screening Programme (see Useful Addresses) recommends that if you are under 25, you should be tested annually, or every time you change partners, and you can get this free and confidential test done as part of the NCSP. Because both men and women can carry the infection without showing any symptoms, this is an important test to consider. For those over the age of 25, speak to your GP.

Incompetent cervix

This is the medical term for a cervix which is weak, and may not remain adequately closed throughout pregnancy. The pressure of a growing fetus may cause the cervix to dilate and cause miscarriage, which occurs after the first three months, usually around sixteen weeks. In women where this is a problem it can cause repeated miscarriages, but once diagnosed it is possible to use a purse-string stitch to help keep the cervix closed. This is sometimes referred to as a Shirodkar stitch and is put in place at around fifteen weeks, under either general or epidural anaesthetic. Careful monitoring is necessary during the first five days following this procedure, in case the insertion of the stitch itself stimulates the cervix and causes miscarriage, but after this it stays put until around the thirty-eighth or thirty-ninth week of pregnancy.

For many women this is all that is needed, but for some the one stitch is not enough. Recent work done by consultant obstetrician Peter Wardle, at St Michael's Hospital, Bristol, to tackle this problem has found that in these women, subsequent monitoring and additional stitches during the course of the pregnancy kept the cervix securely closed until the baby could be safely born. This might mean, for example, a first stitch at around thirteen weeks, followed by another at nineteen weeks, and a last at twenty-three weeks, followed by bed rest. For each woman on whom this technique was tried, the result was a healthy baby born after a series of mid-term miscarriages.

Physical abnormalities of the womb

While around 20% of women experience fibroids, a non-cancerous muscular and fibrous growth on the wall of the womb, very few women have problems with them in pregnancy. However, if there is a history of miscarriage, and a woman has a large fibroid, then its removal is usually advised. If a woman does have fibroids and they are large, they are more likely to be diagnosed beforehand, because they may have played some part in problems with conception.

Fibroids can be diagnosed by taking an abdominal X-ray (if not pregnant), using ultrasound scanning, or hysteroscopy. The hystero-scope is a thin tube with a fibre-optic lens and light source, passed into the womb via the vagina and cervix, which allows the doctor to closely examine the womb lining for abnormalities, including fibroids.

If fibroids are diagnosed, and thought large enough to prevent a pregnancy from continuing successfully, they can be removed under general anaesthetic in an operation called a myomectomy. Subsequent to this, pregnancy will be closely monitored, because some scarring to the lining of the womb may remain.

A very rare condition that may cause miscarriage in the women in which it should occur, is an irregularly shaped womb. This irregularity of shape may mean that, as the fetus grows in the womb, there is not enough room for the pregnancy to continue successfully. If this is the case then a late miscarriage may occur between fourteen and twenty-eight weeks, although many women with oddly-shaped wombs do not have any problem at all.

Surgical correction may solve the problem. Wherever there has been surgery of this scale to the womb, subsequent pregnancies need close monitoring and it may be recommended that the baby is delivered before its due date by caesarean section.

EMOTIONS

No one expects a woman who has miscarried to feel anything but a degree of loss and grief. The time when miscarriage was thought to be just another aspect of a woman's medical lot, and something she was required to 'get over' as soon as possible, has long past. And the expectation that the same feelings of loss can affect the father of the unborn child too, are now recognised as well. The existence of miscarriage support groups bear witness to the necessary process of grieving and eventual acceptance that follows miscarriage. Grief often creates feelings of deep isolation, and here the support of someone who really does have first-hand experience of miscarriage can be invaluable in working through individual feelings.

There is also no evidence to show that stress or anxiety are causative factors in miscarriage. The idea that a sudden shock can make a woman lose her baby is often cited, usually in fiction of the more romanticised kind, but this is unlikely to be the case unless the woman was likely to miscarry anyway. Unborn babies survive all sorts of maternal traumas, both emotional and physical, with no bad effect.

What is remarkable however, is that one single thing that can make a difference to a woman not miscarrying, where she has a history of miscarriage for no apparent reason, is the availability of unconditional loving support: that old-fashioned thing, tender loving care (TLC). Professor Lesley Regan, a UK consultant gynaecologist and obstetrician has delivered medical papers on just this subject. She has conclusive statistical evidence to show that the availability of support from the staff in her miscarriage clinic improves the success rate of subsequent pregnancies in women who have previously miscarried, quite substantially. It seems that simple, reiterated reassurance is more potent than might reasonably be expected given these circumstances.

'I knew that my chances of miscarrying again were unlikely. I knew that this next pregnancy had every chance of being successful. I knew all this rationally, but I just didn't dare to believe it. I really needed the positive voice from the nurse at the clinic to counteract the negative voice in my head. The more I tried not to think about it, the more pervasive the negative voice became! So just to be able to drop in, or ring up and off-load whatever particular anxiety was free-floating around my head was wonderful. I think it helped my husband too: before, when I worried about things and asked him what he thought, it made him feel anxious because he didn't know the answer, or how to reassure me. Now I feel reassured, confident and more in control of events. It makes such a difference.'

Irina, aged 32

PREGNANCY AFTER MISCARRIAGE

Whether you have had one miscarriage or several, whether you know the reasons why miscarriage occurred or not, your next pregnancy and its outcome will quite naturally concern you. It will make no difference if you are told not to worry, because that is inevitable.

It is also possible, however, to help yourself by finding out all you can about why miscarriage might have occurred, positive thinking, harnessing your resources and minimising the fear that you will miscarry again. Look at the statistics and know that the majority of women who miscarry go on to have healthy babies.

Have a good, general, look at your overall health and at a checklist that includes your diet, level of exercise, rest and relaxation, for example (see chapter four, Fit to conceive?). Ask your GP, or Well-Woman clinic for a check-up. Some health authorities run pre-conception clinics where you can talk through your anxieties and receive specialist advice.

One charitable body who have a network of contacts nationwide, is Foresight, the Association for the Promotion of Pre-Conceptual Care (see Useful Addresses). Over the years Foresight has been responsible for supporting research, and making available its findings, into numerous areas concerned with pre-conceptual care, pregnancy and birth. For example, the University of Surrey carried out research that showed the following benefits of the Foresight programme on miscarriage. Where both partners followed the programme, the results showed the following: '. . . of 367 couples, there was a previous miscarriage rate of 83% among the 59% who had had a previous problem pregnancy. By the end of the study 96% of couples in the full study had given birth, without any problems during the pregnancy.'

There is also some evidence to suggest that trace mineral deficiencies can contribute to the incidence of miscarriage. Research that monitored the levels of magnesium and selenium in the blood of a number of women with histories of infertility or early miscarriage, showed encouraging results when their body levels were normalised with supplementation. Other studies show that decreased zinc, or increased copper levels, may have an impact on women who are susceptible. This is not to say that self-prescribing large quantities of minerals or vitamins is the answer, but finding out if this may be a contributing factor can be useful. Again, Foresight is a good organisation to contact for further advice and information.

You may also want to consider some alternative and complementary therapies to increase your vigour and rebalance your energies, covered previously in chapter seven. While none of these approaches could, for example, prevent an inevitable miscarriage if there is a completely random reason for it, feeling strong, calm and positive about yourself before you start, and during the first few weeks when you may feel most anxious about your risk of miscarriage, can only be beneficial.

'It was after the last miscarriage – I had had three – that I took up yoga. I really felt the need to find some strength inside me, and I thought that this would help as well as getting fitter, and concentrating my mind on my body in a more positive way. It also helped me feel as if, by concentrating on my body, it was less alien to me, after having let me down, as I saw it. It also helped that my yoga teacher was quite spiritual, and sympathetic to my particular psychological needs at that time. She also runs a class for pregnant women, which I hope I will transfer to in time!'

Robyn, aged 29

10 Pregnancy

'I was so excited when I saw that thin blue line in the dipstick of the pregnancy test. It seemed such an extraordinary thing, that I should be having a baby! You'd never have thought that millions of women had done it before me!'

Judith, aged 31

'When the result was positive, instead of thinking, how wonderful, my heart sank. I was so afraid something would go wrong, I didn't dare feel optimistic about it. It was weeks before I could allow myself to believe that I was actually going to have a baby – and I didn't feel like celebrating until I saw the scan. It made it very hard on Bob, because I just didn't want anyone to know for a bit.'

Lucy, aged 29

'It was such a relief to get pregnant. I felt as if I could get on with my life now, although in reality I knew nothing would ever be the same again!'

Tricia, aged 35

Whether or not conception has been a long-drawn out battle or a relatively straightforward process, discovering that you are pregnant invariably brings about mixed emotions. Relief, euphoria, fear and excitement are all normal reactions, whatever your situation, because a positive pregnancy test is just the first step and problems can still arise. So it is hard to relax and actually believe that this pregnancy is going to result in a healthy baby in nine months time. The individual, and very personal, experience of getting pregnant will quite naturally colour how you adjust to being pregnant.

Women with a history of infertility, and in particular those who have conceived through IVF and other reproductive technologies, plus those who have experienced miscarriage either once or repeatedly, may quite naturally begin their pregnancies with less confidence than others. Conception, and pregnancy, is already something that has potent psychological overtones connected to the idea of failure, and this may influence ideas about how pregnancy should be managed physically. Having had a lot of involvement with medical expertise, many women find that once pregnancy occurs they feel rather abandoned. However, an IVF pregnancy, once confirmed, is just like any normal pregnancy. It also means it carries much the same risks of miscarriage or ectopic pregnancy, for example. But with so much invested in the pregnancy before it occurs, any subsequent problems can seem much greater, which can be hard to keep in perspective. Although with each passing day and week as pregnancy continues, it becomes easier to feel confident that all is going well.

There is no doubt that pregnancy, under any circumstances, has the potential for increasing stress and anxiety – however much the event is also a cause for celebration and happiness. The impact on a couple's relationship can be profound, and can shake up the assumptions on which it may be based. While some couples find that the whole process draws them together and strengthens their relationship, others find that the tensions that can arise are almost too difficult to solve alone. Negotiating feelings of hope and fear, while trying to get on with day-to-day living, can be very hard. Many infertility centres offer the opportunity for counselling for couples undergoing treatment and it is a facility that should be taken advantage of if available. Otherwise it may be sensible to seek help and support independently, or from one of the specialist charities, for example, the British Infertility Counselling Association (see Useful Addresses), who will also be aware of the continued anxieties that arise even after conception has occurred.

'He was so full of the baby this, the baby that, and kept coming home with things for the baby, that I began to feel like some great seed pod for his offspring. I know it was his way of trying to be involved, but he nearly drove me mad. In the end we had an enormous row but managed to clear the air. Needless to say, it got better after that!'

Angela, aged 37

One of the problems couples may find after a long period of trying to get pregnant, with or without medical help, is that it is difficult to get back to normal after pregnancy is confirmed. It is almost as if the pregnancy alone was the sole goal, rather than a transitional stage on the way to becoming parents. In one way nothing will ever be 'normal' again, as having a baby brings about enormous, and relevant, changes and this is the same for everyone. But where so much has been invested into the possible birth of a baby, the context is slightly different.

It is quite characteristic for women, facing the physical reality of their pregnancy day by day, to become very absorbed and preoccupied by it. The extent of this will be influenced, in part, by their experience of conceiving and, where this has been difficult, the internalised anxiety may make a woman very preoccupied. It is as if she dare not stop thinking about it, in case by letting go emotionally she may somehow let go physically and lose the baby. This preoccupation may mean excluding her partner in some way that has not happened before and this newly intrusive component to the relationship needs some readjustment, which may take time. In addition, if physical concerns and worries mean a woman feels less like being sexually intimate, it is all too easy for feelings of rejection, alienation and resentment to escalate. Suddenly this longed-for baby becomes the reason for all sorts of tensions that did not seem to exist before. Working out what may be a normal reaction to a sequence of events can be difficult, so keeping open lines of communication, while a cliché, is imperative while trying to chart these unknown waters.

'I know John felt that, now I was actually pregnant, he was somehow redundant. It was partly because I felt so sick and irritable during the first few months and, way down deep, I felt he was partly to blame. It was as if this baby, which we had wanted and planned together, was coming between us. It wasn't him feeling like death day in, day out, and I resented it. Luckily we were able to talk about how we felt and, after the first few months adjusting to it all, things settled down.'

Sara, aged 32

TESTING FOR PREGNANCY

Urine tests

The simplest way to test for pregnancy is to use a test manufactured for use at home, bought from the chemist. These urine tests are considered to be 99% accurate under laboratory conditions, but following the instructions closely at home will be good enough! These tests can be used from the first day of a missed period, and although they say that any urine sample is fine, first thing in the morning means that the concentration of pregnancy hormone in the urine is greater.

Alternatively a pregnancy test can be arranged through your GP surgery or health centre, or family planning clinic. You will need to collect a sample of urine first thing in the morning in a clean container, to take to your doctor or clinic. Results usually take twenty-four to forty-eight hours. Remember to ask how you will be told, whether you need to ring or come in to pick up the results.

The pregnancy hormone these tests check for is human chorionic gonadotrophin (HCG). Although this hormone starts being produced by the embryo within seven days of fertilisation, it takes another seven days or so before there is enough produced to make its detection in a urine sample possible.

It is possible to get a false negative test, perhaps because the test was used before the HCG was of sufficient concentration, or because the urine was a very dilute sample, and the instructions then recommend that it is repeated several days later. A false positive test is unlikely: if the test is positive, then there is little doubt that conception has occurred. Pregnancy tests are unaffected by any medication you might be taking, even including the contraceptive pill!

Blood tests

There is available a highly-sensitive blood test for HCG, which can discern whether conception has occurred before a period is due. However this is not usually offered, unless perhaps you have been on an IVF programme, and even then it may not be available as this depends on the policy of the treatment centre. The level of HCG present in the blood is measured, and this can vary. For example, if it is low it may indicate that although fertilisation has occurred, implantation in the lining of the womb may be delayed, or not happening. So specific interpretation of the results may not always be possible at this very early stage and a re-test may be advised. Because of the specialist nature of this blood test, you should have the opportunity to talk through the possible indications of different levels of HCG in the blood with the doctor supervising your treatment.

'Although I was elated when the hospital rang to say that the blood tests showed a raised HCG level, I knew better than to feel too positive until later, when they stayed high and it was safe to presume conception had occurred. It was the most difficult couple of weeks of my life, and if I hadn't had the support of my partner and family, it would have been impossible.'

Grace, aged 33

SIGNS AND SYMPTOMS OF PREGNANCY

Many women, both those who have been pregnant before and those who have not, get a definite feeling that they are pregnant before any test has confirmed it. Equally, other women have no idea and cannot quite believe the reality of the thin blue line on the window of their pregnancy test dipstick. It is completely individual. However, among the physical changes of early pregnancy commonly experienced by women are the following symptoms:

- ◆ swollen, tender breasts, similar to the feeling often experienced prior to a period;
- ◆ a general feeling of nausea which may just occur at a specific time of day, or be ever-present for the first three months;
- ◆ vomiting, which may accompany the nausea;
- ◆ an almost overwhelming sense of tiredness;
- ◆ feeling very emotional and tearful;
- ◆ wanting to pee more frequently than usual;
- ◆ increased sensitivity to different smells and tastes.

If you have one or more of these symptoms, and have missed a period, then it is likely that a pregnancy test will confirm that you have conceived.

'I felt such a fool when I went to the doctor saying I thought I was pregnant and it turned out that I was nearly three months' pregnant . . . No wonder I'd been feeling a little bit under the weather. My periods were always a bit iffy, so I hadn't been sure and I had been too busy to keep a tab on dates, etc. So even thought my home test was positive, I got a shock when the doctor told me how pregnant I probably was!'

Bridie, aged 32

'The nausea was overwhelming. I had always thought pregnancy sickness was 'all in the mind', or some sort of affectation of a Victorian kind. But it hit me with a vengeance: if I hadn't known I was pregnant, I would have thought I was seriously ill. Thank God it passed at around sixteen weeks.'

Emma, aged 28

Many women feel very ambivalent about advertising the fact of their pregnancy for the first few months, apart from sharing the news with their husband or partner, in case the pregnancy fails. This is especially common among those for whom getting pregnant has been a longed-for and difficult process. Not feeling willing to share this news until feeling more confident about the pregnancy continuing is entirely personal, and waiting until after the first three months, for example, to tell people other than immediate family is a sensible option. Although it might mean that should the pregnancy fail no one knows of the particular grief experienced, it does also mean that you avoid well-meaning but hurtful comments when feeling particularly sensitive.

SEEING YOUR DOCTOR

Unless there are specific medical reasons why telling your doctor is important immediately you know you are pregnant, for women with no previous infertility or gynaecological problem there is no need to rush off straight away. Many doctors will do little but congratulate you and give you some general leaflets to read during the first three months, unless you have something in your medical history that suggests closer supervision. However, seeing your doctor earlier rather than later, within the first eight weeks of pregnancy, does mean that you get into the system for antenatal care in good time.

Antenatal care

Antenatal care works on the assumption that pregnancy is a normal event but these regular checks to the mother's health and baby's development ensure that should any problems arise, medical care can be provided in good time. For example, anaemia – where the red blood cells' ability to transport oxygen around the body is limited – is seldom life-threatening but can be easily rectified if picked up during a routine blood test. While iron supplements are seldom given routinely now, they are available if a woman needs them.

Antenatal visits pan out roughly as follows:

- around six weeks, referral by doctor for antenatal care;
- between eight and twelve weeks, first antenatal or 'booking-in' visit;
- antenatal appointments every four weeks until thirty-two weeks pregnant;
- then every two weeks until the baby is delivered.

The booking-in visit is designed to record some baseline health details, but is also your first opportunity to discuss not only issues about where you want to give birth, but also what sort of antenatal tests are relevant to you. Take your time to gather as much information as you can and remember, you seldom have to make decisions now, at this early stage, that cannot be changed later.

In the UK, most antenatal care is offered as 'shared care'. Antenatal care is shared between the community midwives' clinic or GP at your local health centre, and the hospital's obstetric department's antenatal clinic. You may have your first booking-in visit there, after which you see the midwife at the local health centre up to a certain number of weeks. This may mean that out of around ten antenatal visits over your pregnancy, you are seen at the hospital clinic two or three times and the rest of the time by a midwife at the GP surgery or health centre. For women without any complications arising from their pregnancy or past medical history, this provides more than adequate care.

If you are considered a 'high-risk' pregnancy, your pattern of care may be somewhat different, worked out around your individual needs. High-risk mothers-to-be are defined in a number of ways: past gynaecological or obstetric history, maternal age, multiple pregnancy, and general health. Whatever your situation, antenatal care should provide you with time and attention to your particular concerns and requirements.

ANTENATAL TESTS

This has become quite a big issue now that the number and types of antenatal tests have increased. While many of the tests are quite straightforward ways of monitoring a mother's health, the tests for the health of the baby, and whether there may be any congenital abnormalities, are more complex. This is partly because some of the tests carry slight risks themselves, and when a baby is very much longed-for and awaited, balancing up these various risk factors is difficult.

'Although I was prepared to have the baseline tests, I really didn't want a battery of supposedly "routine" tests for congenital disorders . . . but I had to argue against them at every turn. I'm sure the staff thought I was some sort of alternative fanatic, but it was just that I didn't want my pregnancy turned into some sort of reproductive minefield.'

Joanna, aged 27

'I was delighted that my hospital offered a full range of antenatal testing – I had everything going and it meant that, for me, I felt entirely confident of my antenatal care all the way through.'

Yasmin, aged 29

Generally speaking, antenatal tests can be loosely divided into those that are offered routinely and those that are more specific. It is customary in most obstetric practices in the UK to offer the following tests routinely:

- blood tests for blood group, rhesus type and haemoglobin levels;
- blood test to check rubella status;
- blood tests to screen for the levels of a number of substances in the mother's blood which may indicate an increased risk of spina bifida and/or Down's syndrome;
- ultrasound screening.

The first blood test outlined above is a straightforward check on the mother's blood, and self-explanatory. The second check for rubella status should confirm immunity following either having German measles or having had the vaccination as a child (since the measles, mumps and rubella (MMR) vaccines was introduced in 1988, it is now offered routinely to all babies at around thirteen months old). If, for some reason, this check shows no immunity to rubella then it is important to avoid the illness, now becoming more and more infrequent, or to alert the doctor if there has been some known risk of contracting it.

The third blood test outlined is usually done between sixteen to eighteen weeks, following a confirmation of dates from an ultrasound scan. This test is usually the Triple test (sometimes referred to as the Bart's test). The triple test looks at the levels of three substances in the mother's blood: alpha fetoprotein (AFP), human gonadotrophin (HCG) and unconjugated oestriol (uE3). Analysis of these can indicate whether there is an increased *risk* of either spina bifida or Down's syndrome. It is important to understand that, by looking at the levels of particular substances, a risk indicator can be assessed – but this is not the same as a definite diagnosis.

Whether or not you are offered further testing, which will confirm or deny the risk analysis, is both up to an analysis of other known risk factors and whether or not you want to have further testing.

Blood testing is not the only way of assessing risk. The age of the mother has a bearing, and this may be of more relevance to women who have waited a long time to conceive a baby, with or without medical help. For example, the risk factors for Down's syndrome linked to maternal age are as follows:

Your age	Your risk
25	1:1,351
30	1:910
35	1:384
38	1:189

Your age	Your risk
40	1:112
48	1:16

Bear in mind that these statistics are influenced by a number of factors, including the fact that the majority of babies are born to women in their twenties, so the statistics automatically go up for older women purely because less women of this age are having babies. Also, even if your risk factor is 1:1,500 at the age of twenty-five, the risk, still exists. And statistics also show that over 60% of babies with Down's syndrome are born to mothers under the age of thirty-five.

'Aged forty I knew there would be pressure on me to have a battery of tests to see whether the baby I was carrying had Down's syndrome. I knew I had a 1% risk, just based on my age alone but when my blood test showed that I had a risk factor of one in 800, I decided not to have an amniocentesis. After all, I had the same risk factor of a thirty-year-old woman, who wouldn't have been offered anmio anyway. And my baby was fine.'

Patsy, aged 42

So it is in the combination of blood test results, mother's age, ultrasound scan results and exact length of the pregnancy, that a final risk assessment can be arrived at. Also taken into account will be any other known medical factors, for example, previous history of congenital abnormalities, a long-standing condition like diabetes, or if you are carrying more than one baby. So interpretation of results is entirely individual and specific to personal circumstances.

You may, as a woman of thirty-eight have a supposed risk factor of having a baby with Down's syndrome of 1:180, but your blood test may show that there is less of a risk at 1:300. You may be offered amniocentesis just because you are over thirty-seven, but you also know that there is a risk of miscarriage of between 1:100 and 1:250 depending on the hospital that carries out this technique. Your ultrasound scan may show no evidence of the 'soft signs' (see p. 169) of Down's syndrome, so you may, with all the information available decide that further diagnostic testing with amniocentesis is not for you.

If you do proceed to have an amniocentesis, be aware that there will probably be some assumption made about what you want should the test diagnose Down's syndrome. Most people assume that you are taking the test not just because you want to know, conclusively, whether or not your baby is OK but also because if there is a problem, then you would want the pregnancy terminated. Bearing in mind that amniocentesis, following other preliminary assessments of risk factors, may not be possible until between eighteen to twenty weeks of pregnancy, and results take anything up to a maximum of five weeks, then the pregnancy is considerably advanced. Termination would then mean the delivery of a recognisable baby. Termination following diagnosis of abnormality is a particularly difficult dilemma for any woman, but if this is a baby that has been longed-for and tried-for over many years, it is even more difficult. One support group who may be able to offer advice and counselling is ARC – Antenatal Results and Choices (see Useful Addresses).

ULTRASOUND

The use of ultrasound scanning has revolutionised some aspects of antenatal care. It is a particularly useful tool for the diagnosis of multiple pregnancy or placenta praevia (where the position of the placenta blocks the birth canal), it can be used to confirm the gestational age of a baby, and it makes tests like amniocentesis possible. It can also be particularly reassuring in cases of threatened miscarriage where the tangible evidence of a beating heart helps restore a mother's confidence.

Most women accept the routine offer of a first ultrasound scan, to confirm their dates at around sixteen weeks prior to a triple test blood test, without further thought. It must, however, be remembered that ultrasound screening can pick up a number of possible abnormalities in the fetus, and what starts out as a routine checking of dates can become the first step on the road to extensive antenatal testing. For example, if this first scan showed the possibility of an increased thickening of the fold of skin behind the fetus' neck, the 'soft signs' which may be an indication of some chromosomal anomaly, you may find that suggestions are made about further screening with a Nuchal translucency scan, which measures a layer of fluid at the back of the baby's neck. If this shows up thicker than average, amniocentesis likely to be recommended to make a diagnosis.

'I went for my ultrasound scan – just to check my dates – with perfect confidence. Thank goodness I had suggested to Tom that he come too, just to see the baby, because when the technician said he thought there was a problem with the baby, I was very glad not to be on my own. It turned out that he thought the fold of skin at the back of the baby's neck was too thick, and might indicate Edward's Syndrome [a chromosomal problem similar to Down's Syndrome]. They were suggesting amniocentesis to confirm a diagnosis. I'm a Catholic and a termination would be out of the question, so I didn't want the amniocentesis. But I also didn't want to spend the whole of my pregnancy worrying. Instead I had another scan, this time with a specially trained and more experienced doctor. She was very reassuring, and said she was almost 100% confident that I had nothing to worry about. As it turned out, she was right.'

Rachel, aged 33

The reason that this issue is raised here at all is just as a reminder that ultrasound scanning checks for more than just the age of the developing fetus, the position of the placenta and whether or not there is more than one baby. Depending on the skill and expertise of the scan operator it can be used quite conclusively to diagnose certain problems. In itself, this is undoubtedly a good thing, but not if you were unaware of its potential and any additional information comes as a shock.

MULTIPLE PREGNANCY

This is the broad definition for the development of more than one baby in the womb following conception. Pregnancy with twins occurs in around 1% of naturally occurring pregnancies in the UK, while naturally occurring triplets occur once every 8–9,000. Naturally occurring twins can be either identical (also referred to as mono-zygotic or uniovular), which is where the fertilised egg splits in two at an early stage of cell division and both developing babies share the same placenta; or they can be non-identical (dizygotic or biovular) where two eggs were fertilised by two sperm. Identical twins are a random occurrence, while non-identical twins are both more com-mon and can result from a genetic, inherited tendency to conceive twins. Where a woman has conceived among her children a pair of non-identical twins, any daughter she has may subsequently do so too.

'There is no history of twins in my family, and it never occurred to me that I might conceive twins. Consequently it was a huge shock when I went for my sixteen-week ultrasound to have twins diagnosed. It immediately shot me into a high-risk pregnancy category, which was a bit of a blow. I had expected to sail through and work up to the end: no way, by thirty-five weeks I felt bloated, and desperate to deliver.'

Wendy, aged 26

'Having twins was just the best present. We had waited so long for a baby, to have two together seemed a blessing. I was expecting a difficult time but, apart from the caesarean delivery, it was plain-sailing. I even managed to breastfeed them both for nearly five months.'

Beccy, aged 35

IVF and the increased use of fertility drugs has increased the incidence of multiple births. With IVF, a number of eggs are fertilised. It is usual to replace two embryos, while some centres replace three, which is also the legal limit defined by the Human Fertilisation and Embryology Authority (HFEA). One of the potential problems with this, and multiple pregnancies occurring through the use of fertility drugs, is that there are specific risks to both mother and baby associated with multiple pregnancies. While these risks are manageable, and good antenatal care and monitoring ensure this is so, multiple pregnancies invariably become high-risk pregnancies. There is less concern about twin pregnancies, but anything above two babies needs close supervision.

Discovering that you are having more than one baby can come as quite a shock to many women, as they and their partners wonder how they will manage. It may be worth contacting the Multiple Births Foundation (see Useful Addresses) at an early stage to benefit from as much support and advice as you can.

Multiple pregnancy has also given rise to the increasing prevalence of selected termination. Medical advice may recommend that with multiple pregnancies of more than two developing fetuses, it may be beneficial to the health of the mother and the remaining fetus or fetuses, to selectively terminate one or more. This is a very difficult dilemma for parents, and careful counselling and consideration of all information available is important. It is particularly difficult because selective termination means that the life of the selected fetus is terminated, but it remains within the womb until delivery with the remaining baby or babies. This is one of the most difficult, and underestimated, aspects of assisted conception and reproductive technologies. We have the means to accomplish great things, but this most difficult of almost all choices, selecting one life over another, is the downside of creating choice.

PREGNANCY AND AFTER

However a woman becomes pregnant, what happens during the following nine months is hardly less of a miracle, as the baby develops and grows in the womb. With so much invested in pregnancy, it is sometimes hard to see pregnancy for the transitional process it is, especially as there seems a whole industry geared to the pregnant woman. The commercialisation and marketing of pregnancy has almost elevated it to cult status, and occasionally billed it as the latest consumer accessory. It may also be difficult at times to believe that there is anything 'normal' about pregnancy, particularly if it has been hard to come by. As a part of the parenting process, nine months is relatively short compared to the lifetime of care that is required subsequently! But it is also a particularly intense and potentially vulnerable time, especially with a first pregnancy, however it was achieved.

There is no doubt that pregnancy engenders a wealth of conflicting emotions, not just in ourselves, but also in those around us. Being open to our feelings about being pregnant, however conception was achieved, is one of the additional benefits of becoming a parent. Pregnancy is the first step in the opening up of a whole new world and should be welcomed as exactly that, the beginning of a lifetime's journey made by you and your child.

11 Afterword

Although this book is entitled *How To Get Pregnant*, inevitably it covers a lot of material relevant to those who find getting pregnant difficult. For almost twenty years the progress made in reproductive technologies has meant that many more couples, who might well have been childless, have become parents. Even though these technologies exist, their availability remains very haphazard, largely dependent on the financial resources of the individual couples seeking treatment.

Sometimes people speak about the right to have a child, and for the right of infertile couples to have a child in particular, when discussion about the availability of services comes up. For a right to be recognised in law, it has to be enforceable. Under these terms, therefore, having a child cannot be regarded as a right in law.

However, as Sandra Dill, Executive Director of ACCESS, Australia's National Infertility Network, and Director and past-President of the International Federation of Infertility Patient Associations, points out, infertile people do have a right of equity of access to appropriate health care services for the medical condition or disease of infertility, just as someone with a different medical problem would enjoy the right of access for treatment. In the UK, the National Infertility Awareness Campaign (NIAC), works to promote greater access to medical treatment and is an umbrella organisation covering a variety of infertility self-help groups like the Infertility Network and the Donor Conception Network.

Although treatment is regulated by the HFEA in the UK, the decision about who pays for treatment rests with each of the individual district health authorities, very few of which provide a full range of treatments on the NHS. Internationally, the situation remains as mixed. For example, in the USA and Australia, each state has its own legislation about assisted conception. In Sweden and Denmark, treating single women isn't allowed while in Australia some states allow it, while others don't. Some countries, like Egypt and Saudi Arabia forbid all forms of assisted conception treatments using donor sperm, donor eggs, donor embryos or surrogacy, while Norway and Japan allow no surrogacy, egg or embryo donation. The storage of frozen embryos also varies: currently it's allowed for an indefinite period in Finland, ten years in the UK, but only two years in Denmark. In the UK, Sweden, Denmark and Norway, new legislation has abolished the anonymity of egg, sperm and embryo donors. The number of embryos implanted is restricted to three in the UK, and limits are also imposed in France, Germany, and Australia, while in Egypt, the US and Japan guidleines specify a limit, but there is no enforcement mechnanism. In Greece and Canada, however, there are currently neither guidelines nor legislation about the number of embryos transferred.

Whatever the situation in an individual country, there will be among those couples trying to conceive, a proportion who never manage to have a baby of their own. Sandra Dill describes her personal experience:

'I became aware of my infertility problem at the age of twenty-eight after two years of marriage. I was referred for a second opinion and began the usual work-up. In the following years, my husband and I endured the well-meaning but thoughtless comments from friends and acquaintances such as:

- it's not the end of the world, it's just that you can't have a child;
- you're lucky – having children is not easy (neither is being in love, but no one advised me to avoid that);
- it's all for the best (I wonder if these people would say that to the parents of a young child with leukaemia).

After five years we were referred for IVF. We had eight IVF treatment cycles, including an IVF miscarriage at fourteen weeks. After fourteen years of investigating various options, my husband and I were forced to confront the reality that we would never have a child.

Nothing had prepared us to live with this eventuality. The death of a dream of becoming a parent, of forming a family, after so much time, energy and other resources had been committed to its realisation, proved to be extraordinarily difficult to live with.

Some critics in the community have questioned the wisdom of our choice and that of other infertile people to pursue our goal of a child through IVF, but sometimes you need to find the courage to attempt things because they are important to you even when success cannot be guaranteed.

The costs have been high for us – emotionally, physically, financially. However, this has been a personal choice and we are grateful to those who have provided the technology which enabled us to make that choice.

All of us make choices about things we would like to pursue in our lives and most of these achievements come at a cost. We are prepared to meet the costs incurred because we believe those goals we choose to pursue are worthwhile. Our choice was to try to have a child.'

Whatever the reasons why having a child has not been possible, it is the case for many thousands of couples each year. And only they can know what it means to them, and what that individual pain and grief entails. To be childless, not out of choice, but involuntarily, is extremely difficult to come to terms with.

For some couples, the possibility of adopting a child may provide them with an alternative way to become parents. Although there are generally less newborn babies available, adoption remains a very real alternative for many couples, and well worth pursuing as an option. While the disappointment of not being able to become biological parents to a child is not to be underestimated, the possibilities of creating a family in an alternative way may be worth exploring.

In the UK, the organisation BAAF, the British Agencies for Adoption and Fostering (see Useful Addresses), is able to provide comprehensive and up-to-date advice and information. The Infertility Network also provides information on adoption.

Because of the decrease in newborn babies available for adoption over recent years, a couple of organisations also well worth contacting are Adoption UK who are a self-help group formed by parents who had successfully adopted children who were considered 'hard to place'; and Oasis (Overseas Adoption Support and Information Service) who can provide information about the procedure for adopting from abroad.

'For me, adoption made sense of everything that we had gone through before. It showed me that my instincts about my need to be a parent were true and valid, and that our choice was justified. And the opportunity to love our children, and be a family, is a wonderful experience.'

Ceri, aged 36

Glossary

Abandoned cycle

When IVF treatment is discontinued after the giving of drugs to stimulate the production and release of an egg, but before a fertilised egg is transferred to the womb.

Abortion

The clinical description of a miscarriage is a spontaneous abortion, where the pregnancy ceases and the womb expels its contents. This can occur for a number of reasons, and at any time up to twenty-four weeks of pregnancy. Doctors also talk about threatened abortion, or inevitable abortion, and in these cases what is described as abortion is understood by most women to mean miscarriage. Many women find the use of the word abortion in this context distressing, partly because for most women abortion has come to mean that defined, medically, as induced abortion, therapeutic abortion or more commonly, termination of pregnancy (TOP).

Adjusted live birth rate

This is individual to a particular clinic's results where the number of successful births per treatment cycle is adjusted to take into account the different types of patient, and their particular reasons for treatment, that the clinic has treated during any one year.

Amenorrhoea

This is the medical discription for the absence of a monthly period, or menstrual bleed. For many women it can be the first symptom of pregnancy. If menstruation has never occurred then it may be referred to as primary amenorrhoea, to differentiate it from secondary amenorrhoea where there has been a history of menstrual bleeding. Secondary amenorrhoea without pregnancy, and as a cause of infertility, will require investigation to establish its cause.

Antenatal care

The medical care and monitoring given to every pregnant woman before the delivery of her baby, it is designed to pick up and avoid problems that might occur before and at the time of the birth.

Billings method

see Natural family planning

Birth rates

see Adjusted live birth rate, Live birth rate

Blastocyst

This is the earliest stage of pregnancy, about a week after conception. The outer layer develops into the placenta, while the inner cells develop into the fetus and amniotic sac.

Cervical Mucus

The secretions produced by the special cells of the neck of the womb, or cervix, that change in amount and consistency during a woman's fertility cycle.

Conception

The fusion of sperm and egg to form a zygote, which then begins to divide as it travels down the Fallopian tube, to form a blastocyst capable of implantation.

Counselling

It is one of the legal requirements of a licensed clinic that it provide an appropriate counselling service to give clients receiving treatment the chance to talk through all the implications of any treatment they might be considering. It is also available as a resource during treatment designed to provide emotional support to a couple, and to help them cope with any outcome of their treatment.

Donor insemination (DI)

The use of donor sperm to enable a woman to become pregnant when her partner's sperm is incapable of fertilising an egg. Here, the donor sperm is placed inside the woman's vagina or womb mechanically, using a syringe.

Egg collection

Prior to IVF, after a course of drugs to enhance follicle stimulation and ovulation, eggs are collected from a woman's ovaries. Sometimes called egg retrieval.

Embryo

Descriptive term used for the developing baby during the first eight weeks following conception.

Embryo freezing

Embryos, not required for treatment, can be frozen and stored for future use. Also known as cryopreservation, the length of time for which embryos can be legally stored is five years.

Embryo transfer

This is the process by which one or more, but no more than three, embryos are placed in the uterus in the hope that implantation will occur and the woman becomes pregnant.

Endocrinology

A medical specialisation concerning itself with the endocrine system. It is the glands of the endocrine system which secrete hormones, so an endocrinologist is a doctor with additional training and expertise in hormonal problems, which can include working on hormonal issues associated with problems with conception.

Fallopian tubes

Sometimes referred to as the oviducts, but more commonly known by the name of the man who identified them, the Fallopian tubes link the womb to the ovaries, and it is via the Fallopian tube that an egg finds its way to the womb.

Fetus

After eight weeks following conception, the developing embryo is called a fetus.

Follicle

Small sac in the ovary in which the egg develops and which bursts to release the egg at ovulation.

Follicle stimulating hormone (FSH)

The hormone secreted by the pituitary gland responsible for stimulating the ovarian follicle to ovulation.

Gonadotrophin

This is any hormone that has a stimulating effect on the gonads, for example follicle stimulating hormone (FSH) and luteinising hormone (LH) in the female, produced by the pituitary gland.

Gonads

These are the organs responsible for the production of sperm (the testes in the male) and ova (the ovaries in the female).

Infertility

This is the inability to conceive a child. Primary infertility describes the inability to conceive at all, while secondary infertility means that there has been a past history of conception, with or without a successful outcome to the pregnancy. Subfertility is where a couple have been trying for more than a year to conceive.

Insemination

This is the introduction of semen into the womb via the vagina and cervix. Natural insemination occurs through sexual intercourse, but artificial insemination describes the mechanical introduction of semen usually through the use of a syringe.

Intra cytoplasmic sperm injection (ICSI)

A single sperm is injected via the cell wall of the egg into its centre. If fertilisation of the egg occurs, the embryo is then transferred to the womb for possible implantation and pregnancy.

Intra uterine insemination (IUI)

Here the sperm is placed inside the womb, inserted mechanically via the cervix, rather than just into the vagina.

In-vitro fertilisation (IVF)

Eggs collected from a woman are mixed with the man's sperm in a sterile container. If fertilisation takes place, one or more (but no more than three) embryos are placed in the womb in the hope that they will implant and pregnancy occurs.

Laparoscopy

Examination of the interior of the abdomen using a laparoscope, a fibre-optic tube enabling the doctor to look into the abdominal cavity through a small incision and examine the internal organs.

Live birth

This is the safe delivery of one, or more, live babies.

Live birth rate

The number of live births that have resulted from every 100 treatment cycles started, and recorded by a clinic.

Luteinising hormone (LH)

Once FSH has produced a mature ovarian follicle, LH is responsible for actual ovulation, and the development of the corpus luteum which will secrete progesterone. In the male, LH is responsible for stimulating the development of cells in the testes that secrete testosterone.

Menstrual Cycle

Also referred to as the female fertility cycle, this lasts around twenty-eight days, although each woman's cycle length is individual to her. This cycle consists of the release of an egg from the ovary (ovulation), the preparation of the lining of the womb in case fertilisation and implantation occurs, followed by the loss of blood and tissue via the vagina if this does not occur.

Miscarriage

The loss of a pregnancy any time from conception to twenty-four weeks. Also referred to, medically, as a spontaneous abortion.

Motility

When applied to sperm, this describes their ability to move.

Mucus

see Cervical Mucus

Multiple birth

This is the birth of more than one baby at a time, twins or triplets or more. However, each multiple birth is counted as a single live birth in statistics recorded by a clinic.

Multiple pregnancy

This is a pregnancy where more than one fetal heartbeat is detected.

Natural family planning (NFP)

This is based on the use of an individual woman's awareness of her own fertility cycle, and when she ovulates, to either avoid or enhance her chances of conception. Using a number of fertility indicaters – basal body temperature charting, mucus symptoms, feel of the cervix, and mid-cycle pain, for example – which a woman has been taught to recognise, a couple can use this information to plan their family. In Australia this is often referred to as the Billings Method, after a Dr Billings who first described and taught the technique.

Neonatal death

The death of a baby within twenty-eight days of delivery.

Oestrogen

A hormone secreted by the ovary, in response to the stimulation of FSH and LH, prior to ovulation.

Ova

Plural of ovum, meaning a number of eggs.

Ovulation

The release of a mature ovum or egg, capable of fertilisation, from the ruptured follicle of the ovary.

Pregnancy rate

This is a record of the number of pregnancies achieved from every 100 treatment cycles started. This is a different statistic to the live birth rate.

Progesterone

Hormone secreted by the corpus luteum, the ruptured follicle that remains after ovulation, and responsible for the thickening of the womb lining in preparation for possible implantation. If implantation does occur, the corpus luteum continues to secrete progesterone until the development of the placenta is mature enough to take over its production to sustain the pregnancy, at about twelve weeks.

Prolactin

After a baby is born, this hormone is secreted by the pituitary gland to stimulate milk production in the breasts. Breastfeeding a baby, and in particular the baby's sucking, stimulates a continued supply of prolactin, so ensuring a continued supply of milk. A sustained level of prolactin prevents secretion of FSH and LH, so prevents further ovulation. Sometimes prolactin is secreted by the pituitary gland in other circumstances, perhaps because of the presence of a benign pituitary tumour causing a degree of pressure. This can sometimes be a cause of infertility, picked up by blood testing or skull X-ray.

Secondary infertility

See Infertility

Semen

This is what appears at male ejaculation and consists of seminal fluid from the prostate gland and sperm produced by the testes.

Sperm

This is the male reproductive cell, the counterpart to the femal ovum. Sperm are produced continuously from puberty to old age, in the testes, in large quantities and are expelled at ejaculation within the seminal fluid.

Stillbirth

This is a baby born after the twenty-fourth week of pregnancy who has not breathed at all, or shown any other sign of life, after having been expelled from its mother's body. Such a baby requires a Stillbirth Certificate to be made out by a doctor or registered midwife present at the birth, so the baby's birth can be registered prior to its burial or cremation.

Subfertility

See Infertility

Superovulation stimulation

Through the use of a particular drug regime, a woman's ovaries are stimulated to produce more eggs than usual in one monthly cycle. This is often done prior to egg collection for IVF to allow for a number of embryos to be produced at one time.

Surrogate mother

Woman who carries a baby, usually the result of an IVF conception, in her womb throughout pregnancy until birth, for another woman. The baby is genetically not hers, and the understanding is that the baby will be born in this way on behalf of its biological parents.

Testosterone

Male sex hormone responsible for the production of sperm in the testes and the development of secondary sex characteristics (deepening voice, growth of beard, pubic hair, etc.) after puberty.

Test tube baby

Description of a baby born via IVF, where the egg is fertilised by the sperm not in fact in a test tube, but in a sterilised dish.

Treatment cycle

A cycle of treatment can vary, depending on the three main treatments used. It could be an IVF cycle using fresh embryos; an IVF cycle using previously frozen embryos; or a DI cycle using donor sperm for insemination. The cycle begins with any necessary preparation of an individual woman's body to make implantation more likely, and continues until the cycle is completed either by a menstrual period where pregnancy has not occurred, of with a positive diagnosis of pregnancy itself.

Zygote

The fertilised ovum, prior to the cell division that creates the blastocyst prior to becoming an embryo and capable of implantation.

Useful addresses

ACCESS (Australia)
PO Box 3605
Rhodes
NSW 2138
Australia
02 9737 0158
www.access.org.au

Adoption UK
Linden House
55 The Green
South Bar Street
Banbury
Oxon OX16 9AB
01295 752240
www.adoptionuk.org

AIMS (Association for Improvements in Maternity Services)
5 Ann's Court
Grove Road
Surbiton
Surrey KT6 4BE
0208 390 9534
www.aims.org.uk

ARC (Antenatal Results & Choices)
73 Charlotte Street
London W1T 4PN
Helpline 020 7631 0285
www.arc-uk.org

Biolab Medical Unit
9 Weymouth Street
London WIW 6DB
020 7636 5959/5905
www.biolab.co.uk

BAAF (British Agencies for Adoption & Fostering)
Saffron House
6–10 Kirby Street
London EC1N 8TS
020 7421 2600
www.baaf.org.uk

BACP (British Association for Counselling & Psychotherapy)
BACP House
15 St John's Business Park
Lutterworth
Leicestershire LE17 4HB
01455 883300
www.bacp.co.uk

British Fertility Society
22 Apex Court
Woodlands
Bradley Stoke BS32 4JT
01454 642217
www.fertility.org.uk

British Infertility Counselling Association
01372 451626
www.bica.net

COTS (Childlessness Overcome Through Surrogacy)
Lairg
Sutherland IV27 4EF
www.surrogacy.org.uk

Donor Conception Network
PO Box 7471
Nottingham NG3 6ZR
020 8245 4369
www.dcnetwork.org

Endometriosis UK
50 Westminster Palace Gardens
Artillery Row
London SW19 1RR
020 7222 2781
www.endometriosis-uk.org

Fertility Europe
Rijsenbergstaat 150
9000 Gent
Belgium
www.fertilityeurope.eu

Fertility UK
Bury Knowle Health Centre
207 London Road
Headington
Oxford OX3 9JA
www.fertilityuk.org

Foresight (Association for the Promotion of Pre-Conceptual Care)
178 Hawthorn Road
West Bognor
West Sussex PO21 2UY
01243 868 001
www.foresight-preconception.org.uk

HFEA (Human Fertilisation and Embryology Authority)
21 Bloomsbury Street
London WC1B 3HF
020 7291 8200
www.hfea.gov.uk

Hughes Syndrome Foundation
Louise Coote Lupus Unit
Gassiot House
St Thomas' Hospital
London SE1 7EH
020 7188 8217
www.hughes-syndrome.org

Infertility Network
Charter House
3 St Leonard's Road
Bexhill on Sea
East Sussex TN40 1JA
08701 188088
www.infertilitynetworkuk.com

London Fertility Centre
112a Harley Street
London W1G 7JH
020 7224 0707
www.lfc.org.uk

Maternity Action
Unit F5
89–93 Fonthill Road
London N4 3JH
020 7281 7816
www.maternityaction.org.uk

Miscarriage Association
c/o Clayton Hospital
Northgate
Wakefield WF1 3JS
01924 200799
www.miscarriageassociation.org.uk

Multiple Births Foundation
Queen Charlotte's and Chelsea Hospital
Du Cane Road
London W12 0HS
020 8383 3519
www.multiplebirths.org.uk

National Chlamydia Screening Programme (NCSP)
www.chlamydiascreening.nhs.uk

National Gamete Donation Trust
Confidential helpline 0845 226 2193
www.ngdt.co.uk

National Family Planning Teachers' Association (NFPTA)
www.nfpta.org.uk

Oasis (Overseas Adoption Support and Information Service)
Confidential helpline: 0870 2417 069
www.adoptionoverseas.org

QUIT (Quit smoking)
St Mary's Axe
London EC3A 8AA
020 7469 0400
Quitline 0800 00 22 00
www.quit.org.uk

Relate (The Relationship People)
Premier House
Caroline Court
Lakeside
Doncaster DN4 5RA
0300 100 1234
www.relate.org.uk

Resolve (National Infertility Association USA)
Suite 500
1760 Old Meadow Road
McLean
VA 22102
USA
00 1 703 556 7172
www.resolve.org

Zita West Clinic
37 Manchester Street
London W1V 7LJ
020 7224 0017
www.zitawest.com

ALTERNATIVE THERAPIES

Aromatherapy Council
www.aromatherapycouncil.co.uk

Association of Reflexologists
5 Fore Street
Taunton
Somerset TA1 1HX
01823 351010
www.aor.org.uk

BMAS (British Medical Acupuncture Society)
Royal London Homeopathic Hospital
60 Great Ormond Street
London WC1N 3HR
020 7713 9437
www.medical-acupuncture.co.uk

College of Naturopathic Medicine UK
Unit 1, Bullrushes Farm
Coombe Hill Road
East Grinstead
West Sussex RH19 4LZ
01342 410505
www.naturopathy-uk.com

Complementary Medicine Association
0845 129 8434
www.the-cma.org.uk

Confederation of Healing Organisations
01584 890662
www.confederation-of-healing-organisations.org

Foundation for Paediatric Osteopathy
41 Woodbridge Street
London EC1R 0ND
020 7490 5510
www.fpo.org.uk

General Osteopathic Council
176 Tower Bridge Road
London SE1 3LU
020 7357 6655
www.osteopathy.org.uk

National Institute of Medical Herbalists
Elm House
54 Mary Arches Street
Exeter EX4 3BA
01392 426022
www.nimh.org.uk

Register of Chinese Herbal Medicine
Office 5
1 Exeter Street
Norwich
Norfolk NR2 4QB
01603 623994
www.rchm.co.uk

Shiatsu Society
PO Box 4580
Rugby
Warwickshire CV21 9EL
0845 130 4560
www.shiatsusociety.org

Society of Homeopaths
11 Brookfield
Duncan House
Moulton Park
Northampton NN3 6WL
0845 450 6611
www.homeopathy-soh.com

The Healing Trust
21 York Road
Northampton
NN1 5QG
01604 603247
www.thehealingtrust.org.uk

ADDITIONAL WEBSITES OF INTEREST

www.daisynetwork.org.uk (Premature menopause support group)
www.fertilityfriends.co.uk (Online community of UK infertility patients)
www.foodstandards.gov.uk (UK government information and advice)
www.mothers35plus.co.uk (Information and resources for older mums)
www.nutrition.org.uk (British Nutrition Foundation)
www.repromed.co.uk (Bristol Centre for Reproductive Medicine)
www.sart.org (US Site for Society for Assisted Reproductive Technology)
www.shetrust.org (Advice and information on endometriosis)
www.verity-pcos.org.uk (Information and advice charity for women with polycystic ovary symdrome)
www.womens-health.co.uk (Good information and advice on general women's health)

SUPPLIERS

Ainsworth Pharmacy
38 New Cavendish Street
London W1G 8UF
020 7935 5330
www.ainsworths.com

Glasgow Health Solutions (supplier of pharmaceutical grade Omega 3 EFAs)
Omega House
12 Sovereign Court
Wyrefields
Poulton le Fylde
Lancashire FY6 8JX
0800 027 3807
www.glasgowhealthsolutions.com

Helios Homeopathy
97 Camden Road
Tunbridge Wells
Kent TN1 2QR
01892 537254
www.helios.co.uk

Lumie (Full spectrum lighting)
3 The Links
Trafalgar Way
Bar Hill
Cambridge CB23 8UD
01954 780500
www.lumie.com

Neal's Yard Remedies
Peacemarsh
Gillingham
Dorset SP8 4EU
01747 834634
www.nealsyardremedies.com

Resperate (Relaxation and clinically proven aid to lowering blood pressure)
Forum Business Centre
Lansdown Road
Cheltenham
Gloucestershire GL50 2JA
0800 177 7778
www.resperate.co.uk

Yes® Pure Intimacy (Certified organic fertility friendly lubricant system)
3L Trading
PO Box 214
Alton
Hants GU34 3WY
0845 094 1141
www.yesyesyes.org

Further reading

The Art of the Nap, Harriet Griffey, MQPublications

Diabetes and Pregnancy, Anna Knopfler, Vermilion

Fertility and Conception, Zita West, Dorling Kindersley

Getting Pregnant: The Complete Guide to Fertility and Infertility, Professor Robert Winston, Pan

The Gift of a Child: Artificial Insemination by Donor, Robert and Elizabeth Snowden, University of Exeter Press

Infertility: New Choices, New Dilemmas, Elizabeth Bryan and Ronald Higgins, Penguin

Infertility: Tests, Treatments and Options, Roger Neuberg, Thorsons

Labours of Eve: Women's Experience of Infertility, Katherine Barby, Boxtree

Male Infertility: Men Talking, Mary-Clare Mason, Routledge

A Manual of Natural Family Planning, Dr Anna Flynn and Melissa Brooks, Thorsons

Miscarriage, Professor Lesley Regan, Bloomsbury.

Natural Healing for Women, Susan Curtis and Romy Fraser, Pandora Press

The Fertility Diet, Chavarro/Willett, McGraw Hill Publishers

The Natural Way with Infertility, Belinda Whitworth, Element Books

Pregnancy and Childbirth, Sheila Kitzinger, Michael Joseph

Pregnancy: The Inside Story, Joan Raphael-Leff, Sheldon Press

Preparation for Pregnancy: An Essential Guide, Suzanne Gail Bradley and Nicholas Bennett, Argyll Publishing

The Really Useful A-Z of Pregnancy and Birth, Harriet Griffey, Thorsons

The Subfertility Handbook, Virginia Ironside and Sarah Biggs, Sheldon Press

The Tentative Pregnancy, Barbara Katz Rothman, Pandora Press

The Truth About Hormones, Vivienne Parry, Atlantic Books

Index